MESSAGE IN A BOTTLE

Questions from Parents About Teen Alcohol and Drug Use

Jeff Wolfsberg
with Deborah Drake

WOLFPACK PUBLISHING GROUP

www.JeffWolfsberg.com
© 2012

Message in a Bottle: Questions from Parents About Teen Alcohol and Drug Use

All Rights Reserved. Copyright © 2012 by Wolfpack Publishing

Address inquiries regarding training and volume orders to:
Jeff Wolfsberg and Associates, Inc
Email info@jeffwolfsberg.com or call 425-223-5335

ISBN 13: 978-0-985358402
ISBN-10: 0985358408

Publisher: Wolfpack Publishing Group
Contributor & Editor: Deborah Drake
Cover Design: Julia Madrigan (www.juliamadrigan.com)
Interior Layout: Deborah Drake

The authors have made every attempt to provide accurate information and to properly attribute all sources. Both the authors and publisher have applied their best efforts in the creation of this book. It is sold with the understanding that no one is rendering legal, medical, financial, or any other professional advice or services. Should you require expert advice or services, you should contact a competent professional. No warranties, expressed or implied, are represented, and neither the publisher nor the author shall be liable for any loss of profit or any other financial or emotional damage in the use of this book

Printed in the United States of America

First Edition 2 4 6 8

DEDICATION

To my loving family—Mom, Dad, Jim, John, and Jennifer
All my love and thanks.

ACKNOWLEDGMENTS

To my wife and friend Elenie who has been a constant source of support and love since I was seventeen—thank you.

I'd like to express my sincere thanks to Deborah Drake for breathing life into *Message in a Bottle*. This project has been sitting on my computer for years. Deb's enthusiasm and support brought it to fruition.

Additional thanks to all the schools who have invited me on campus and believe in the mission of healthier teens and communities free of the harm associated with alcohol misuse, drugs, and addiction.

I cannot imagine my life without my great friends Cindy, Laurie, Chris, Zac, Scott, and Chuck for their support and friendship. My admiration and love to my best friend David for many years of friendship and brotherhood. My deep respect and thanks to Sal for his professional support and friendship the last couple of years. I'd like to express my love to my second family, Tina, Paul, Patty, Cynthia, and Nick for their endless and unconditional love and support.

A BIG thank you to Dr. Jane Bluestein for contributing the Foreword. Jane is an amazing educator, friend, and colleague.

A final thanks to the students past and present who have shared their lives with me during my seminars. I have been personally enriched by your courage and proud to have been a guide to your journey of self-exploration.

TABLE OF CONTENTS

Foreward.....*1*

Introduction.....*7*

Defining Terms.....*17*

1 I'm not very knowledgeable about drugs. How could I tell if my child is using drugs?.....*25*

2 If I discover my child is using drugs, what do I do?.....*29*

3 I have one son in the fifth grade and I can already see how intense the peer pressure is getting for him. How can I support him to not give in to it and make decisions for himself?.....*33*

4 My son came home the other day and asked me if I ever did drugs!.....*41*

5 If I suspect my child is using drugs, is it alright for me to snoop in her room?.....*49*

6 I want my son to trust me—yet what should I do when he tells me that a friend of his drinks and uses other drugs?.....*53*

7 Alcoholism runs in our family, when should I tell my kids about it?.....*59*

8 How soon should I begin talking to my kids about alcohol and other drugs?.....*63*

9 What are some of the drug trends today? *67*

10 What do I do if my child has come home drunk?.....71

11 How do I support and encourage my child not to use alcohol and other drugs?.....*75*

12 How do I start a conversation with my daughter about alcohol and drugs?.....*83*

13 How might I teen-proof our house from drugs and alcohol? I'm concerned my teen might take advantage of drinking when I am away.....*87*

14 What do I say to my graduating senior about college next year and all the drinking and partying that I read about in the news?.....*91*

15 Where do kids get the alcohol? And when do kids start drinking or using other drugs?.....*97*

16 Should I allow my son to go to a party where I know there will be drinking?.....*101*

17 I heard the pot smoked today is 10-20 times stronger than the pot that was smoked a generation ago? Is that true?.....*103*

18 I've been to a million of these parent education workshops, but the parents that really need to be here are not. How do we get them to show up?.....*107*

19 Don't you think you are sending the wrong message to kids when you are a recovering person teaching drug education?.....*109*

20 My daughter's prom is coming up. My wife and I are worried about the whole party scene surrounding the prom. What can we do to ensure she has a great time but safely?.....*111*

21 My son is curious about alcohol. Should I sit down with him and allow him to drink until he knows how it feels to be drunk to eliminate the curiosity?.....*115*

22 Is it okay to drink in front of my kids?.....*117*

Some Final Words.....*119*

Just For the Weekend.....*121*

FOREWORD

by Dr. Jane Bluestein, PhD

There's a question that comes up in nearly every interview I've done for the past three decades: "How are kids different today?" Despite the persistent and increasing acceleration in every corner of our culture and technology that has occurred during this time, I find myself offering the same answer each time. Because to be honest, I don't believe that kids are actually that much different from young people in years past. Today's teens have the same basic needs for things like belonging, acceptance, safety, success, worth, autonomy, structure and security, for example, as any child in history. What *has* changed— and changed to an astronomical degree— are the resources and avenues available to young people for getting these needs met.

Now whether you see this avalanche of information, technology, material goods, and communications as a technological nirvana crammed with an abundance of positive opportunities, or as the doorway to Dante's third circle of Hell, it's probably a good idea to make peace with progress and with the breathtaking speed at which it is unfolding. Instead of pining for simpler times (and you'll notice I very deliberately did not call them "good old days"), I think we'll be much better served to point our energies and intentions toward creating relationships and environments to help our kids successfully navigate these increasingly complex and challenging times.

Keep in mind that whether we make a choice impulsively or deliberately, emotionally or analytically, we make our decision to satisfy the need that feels the most important at the time. If finishing a chore takes priority over watching TV or checking email, we hold off on our break until we're finished. If the chore is especially unpleasant, or we haven't had a break for a while, its importance diminishes in light of more attractive options.

For better or worse, drugs and alcohol can be fairly attractive options for young people.[1] And let's face it, anything that kids perceive as an opportunity to feel something pleasurable—much less actually experience—take the edge off stress and anxiety, numb out painful feelings, find acceptance among peers they value, and look cool in the process is a pretty easy sell. (If you've ever stayed up too late to watch TV or play a video game, gone over your budget purchasing a non-essential item, or finished a big dessert you were planning on declining, you know what I'm talking about. Even mature, well-balanced adults don't always make the best decisions from a rational perspective.)

Each choice offers its own payoff, and we always go with the option that promises the best payoff at the moment we decide. Later, we may wish we *had* bought the souvenir or eaten the brownie, but at the moment of decision, we chose to delay gratification in favor of the potentially negative

---

[1] When I talk about drugs and alcohol, I'm also referring to tobacco, food, work or achievement, sex or relationships, gambling, shopping, or any other potentially addictive substance or behavior pattern.

results of the alternative choice, something many teens have difficulty anticipating.

We tell kids that drugs and alcohol are bad, but the fact that these substances offer so many attractive payoffs is what makes them seem good, which is exactly what makes them dangerous. Yes, there are potentially horrible consequences, but to a teen brain—which, from a developmental standpoint, doesn't catch up to the body for several more years— horrible consequences are far more likely to happen to somebody else, or seem too far off in the future to be of any immediate concern.

I think that as long as we concentrate our prevention efforts on making drugs and alcohol look harmful and destructive, we risk tempting kids to test our credibility. We've also seen how ineffective this approach can be, especially for kids who see these substances as an avenue for meeting basic needs, whether they are seeking the safety and comfort of an escape, looking for acceptance and belonging, or competing for power and autonomy, for example.

Perhaps, then, the best way to prevent drug and alcohol use is not to attempt to make the substances or behaviors less attractive, but to make them less *necessary*.

Let's focus on meeting these same needs to whatever degree is possible within the context of our relationships and home (and school) environments, and giving young people the tools they need to make constructive choices when faced with competing and attractive options.

I believe we have a great deal of power to influence many of the factors that color the way kids perceive and interpret the options they have in the choices they encounter. Here are a few things we can do to connect with kids as safe, trustworthy adults, to building skills they'll need when we're not there to tell them what to do, and to creating a safe, structured, and loving environment they don't feel the need to escape.

Love unconditionally. Seemingly from the time they are born, children get countless messages about their conditional value and worth based on their ability to please the adults in their lives. Is it any wonder that so many are vulnerable to the conditional approval of their peers, and willing to make risky decisions to fit in? When your love and acceptance of your children is not expressed as conditionally available depending on their ability to keep their rooms clean, keep their grades up, follow rules, or make you look good, it's easier for them to believe that you really do care about them no matter what.

Accommodate their need for structure and limits. Clear boundaries and good follow through creates a sense of structure, safety and predictability for all concerned. Structure requires clear directions, understandable limits, and a commitment to follow through without giving warnings or asking for excuses.

Motivate without threats. We almost automatically focus on negative consequences, so this may take some practice. Try stating contingencies that emphasize positive outcomes, focusing instead on the benefit to them for doing what you want. "You can have the car when (or if)..." can increase cooperation and reduce opposition you're more likely to encounter with "You can't have the care unless (or if you don't)..." It's subtle, put the shift is powerful.

Appreciate and accommodate their need for power and autonomy within those limits. I've met very few people struggling with addictions who did not also have control issues. Win-win power dynamics will leave you in charge without disempowering your children or robbing them of their need to manage and influence their own lives, much less the need to seek substances or risky behaviors to prove you can't control them.

Build decision-making skills. The majority of hard choices your kids will have to make will occur when you're not around. Decision-making muscle doesn't develop in a vacuum, however, and if you've been giving them choices from a young age, you've probably seen some skill develop in this area. If not, start now, offering them opportunities for them to make decisions—which helps them connect their choices to the outcomes they experience as a result.

Look for teachable moments. Help your children use their mistakes and apparent errors in judgment as opportunities for learning. Rather than blaming or criticizing, try to stay calm and guide them to think through what else they might have done, what might have happened had they made a different choice, and how they might handle a similar situation differently in the future.

Listen. Your kids are more likely to trust you enough to share their thoughts and feelings in an emotionally safe environment where they know they're not likely to encounter a negative response such as impatience, criticism, ridicule, disappointment, restrictions, or punishment. Even advice-giving can be risky because it assumes responsibility for their problem and may, in fact, make things worse, with you to conveniently blame. When you can resist the urge to tell them what to do, asking questions can often guide them to their own solutions, and the sense of competence that comes with it.

Validate the reality of what they are experiencing, even if their reality doesn't make much sense to you, or is very different from how you would respond in that situation. Sometimes simply agreeing with them can reduce the likelihood of being dismissed or having them feel the need to dig in to prove their reality to you.

Take care of yourself. If your behaviors, attitudes, language, and tone of voice aren't modeling what you'd like to see and hear from your children, look for ways to make small changes to get more in line with what you want them to emulate. Get help if necessary.

I'm delighted to provide the Foreword to this wonderful book and look forward to sharing this resource with the parents I encounter in my work. Just as important as the actual answers and explorations this book offers is the context in which these exchanges with your children will occur. Your relationship with your children can be a powerful and protective asset as they navigate the day-to-day challenges, as well as the risks and temptations, they will encounter throughout their lives. And when they ask the tough questions or confront you with difficult situations, as they invariably will, you'll find concrete answers and valuable, practical information in the following pages.

Albuquerque, New Mexico

Jane Bluestein is a speaker and educator and author of numerous books including *Parents, Teens and Boundaries: How to Draw the Line* and *Creating Emotionally Safe Schools: A Guide for Parents and Educators.*

For more about Jane Bluestein and her work visit www.janebluestein.com

INTRODUCTION

At the time of this writing, we are experiencing a thirty-year high in teen alcohol and other drug use. Admissions to drug treatment centers have been escalating for years with young adult admissions at scary levels. Alcohol and marijuana continue to be an ongoing and persistent problem, but the number of young adults entering treatment for narcotics addiction is reaching epidemic levels.

Never in my fifteen years of work have I heard more teens and adults tell me stories of deadly overdoses of friends and family members. Young people, characterized as good young men and women with talent, good families, from good communities, going to excellent schools, dying from overdoses of prescription medication. For me, this is simply unacceptable and I believe that parents want better for their children. And, like in the movie Network—I'm mad as hell and not going to take it anymore.

This slender volume is not intended to be a parenting "how to" book as the title may imply. It is however, a book for parents. If this book is the tenth book on parenting you have bought this year in an attempt to build the perfect child, put it down. You will not find the holy grail of parenting wisdom here. As a matter of fact, I may even frustrate you a little or a lot somewhere along the way as you are reading.

You are about to enter the world of uncertainty, finger-crossed, and deep sighs of relief at the sound of your front door opening at or past curfew, if you have one to enforce.

I do not consider myself a parenting expert though I have a great deal of experience working with teens and their parents. At the time of this writing, I am not even a parent. In part because of my own history, I opted not to become a parent but I am a devoted brother, son, and uncle to my nieces and nephews and as an educator I have worked with thousands of students. I have also worked with parents in a variety of environments including schools, drug treatment centers, and community coalitions. I have spent an enormous amount of time listening to teens talk about their lives and their ideas about drinking, drug use, family and school life, and mental health.

You will find, throughout this book parents, teachers, and students have shared their stories of hope, disappointment, and success transgressing the turbulent waters of adolescence. I am indebted to them for these gifts of story and humbled to have them share them with me.

No parent wants to learn that their teen is drinking or using other drugs. However, statistically speaking, there is a better than good chance your teen will at least try alcohol, marijuana, or other drugs. Will it lead to habitual use, problematic use, abuse, addiction, I don't know.

There is a confluence of factors that come together to create vulnerability. Some are out of your control like genetics and disposition, and others that are in your control like environment and parenting style. Obviously, we will focus on what is in your control.

Whether you are a private school parent or public school parents, city or rural school, there is little chance that your family will be able to avoid alcohol and other drugs. Don't consider alcohol and other drug use as "something you will try to avoid" but rather "it's inevitable and we are going to deal with it early and often."

Personally, I have lost my patience with today's "super" parent and their attempts to create children I experience potentially as achievement monsters. I am not going to bash parents in this book. I do not think parents are to blame for all the teenage drinking and other drug problems. Finger-pointing is part of the problem and there are enough people and things to blame if we wanted to. Adolescents have to be held responsible for their behavior and the choices they make.

There are plenty of cases where an active and engaged parent has a child who is making terrible decisions. That aside, American *parent* culture is infected with the disease of perfectionism and what I call "neglect by abundance."

Perfect parenting is simply not possible. If it were—I'm not sure what it is anyway—it is still not a guarantee that your child will not experiment and potentially become harmfully involved with alcohol or other drugs. Nor does this not mean that parents are helpless bystanders to the pressures and influences surrounding adolescents to drink and use other drugs. Thousands of parents have attended my parent workshops in hopes of hearing the silver bullet of drug-free parenting. No silver bullet exists.

Parents, do the best you can with the tools you have and acknowledge yourself for doing the best you can. Yet, parenting that minimizes the dangers posed by underage drinking and other drug use does not happen by accident.

There is an *abundance* of evidence that has led researchers and practitioners to identify specific attitudes and behaviors that will increase or decrease the likelihood of an adolescent drinking harmfully or using other drugs.

The role of parents in a teen's choice to drink or use other drugs is paradoxical. There is very little parents can do to insulate their children from exposure to underage drinking and other drugs. At the same time, there is much they can do to help and support their children in making positive health affirming choices.

I believe it requires decisions about family life that are counter intuitive to the current cultural messages of what it takes to raise a successful teen. I see a lot of teens who have the external appearance of achievements, adorned with decorations of superiority, but have no connection to their inner lives, are quietly miserable and use chemicals to numb the existential separation that they are experiencing from who they think they are and who the world wants and tells them to be.

What is an antidote? Start with slowing family life down. Doing less allows for connecting more. More is not always more. More is often less: less connection, less love, less vibrancy in family life. I encourage you to just stop. Push the pause button and just listen quietly for the heartbeat of your family. It is funny what shows up in the silence if you allow it. I often ask parents during my workshops to think about a time when they felt their family was thriving, vibrant, and connected. "What were you doing to achieve that? What were the daily practices that led to these outcomes? How can you return to this family "state" and achieve this result over and over again?" I think it is possible.

To be effective requires parents to scrutinize our culture in a way their own parents never had to. Parents must develop the internal resolve to be "temporarily" disliked by their children for making unpopular decisions. It takes courage and wisdom to know the difference between being a friend and a parent. It requires more courage to allow children to be individuals, make mistakes and test family values as they develop their identity.

May you have the courage it takes to let your kids be themselves and test the boundaries. Today's parents need to know how to distance the family from a toxic culture saturated with health-damaging messages—without allowing the family to become isolated, cynical, and out-of-touch.

There are no simple answers to reducing underage drinking and drug use or one answer that works for everyone. The insights expressed in this book are based on my experiences. My experience with parents and students has also been predominantly in working with independent schools. My answers, suggestions, and stories relate to their experience. I do feel that the stories shared in this book transcend many socioeconomic and cultural barriers.

At the end of the day teens in public and private education are facing the same fundamental choices to experiment with alcohol and other drugs or say no with conviction.

There is no shortage of books on raising children. At your local bookstore or online you will find a myriad of options full of parenting advice. There are so many parenting books today I think many parents have become confused and have lost trust in their own intuition.

To complicate matters, some advice contradicts other advice so which experts are we supposed to trust? With the proliferation of parenting books, a parent may assume that an answer to almost any problem is buried somewhere in the thousands of pages of parenting advice written each year. Lost in the deluge of expert advice is the basic idea of trusting your gut and calling it like it is.

I resisted the temptation to write a "7 Steps to a Happy Family" type of book. I don't think there are steps. Titles like that may sell books but they don't make happier families. I have no idea how to tell you to become happy or have a happy family. I didn't grow up in a happy family.

My parents are loving people, but also deeply wounded from their own upbringings. They did the best they could with the tools they had, but their wounds left huge deficits in my own needs as a teen growing up. I had to find my own path towards happiness. I'm still looking. I can tell you where it is not found, which represents a big part of my work with students.

May this book supports you in reconnecting with your intuition and empowers you to call it like it is. I believe the primary task of parents is to keep their children alive until they can do the game of life on their own. Effective parenting begins with getting your child to the age where they can support themselves without a life destroying addiction.

The format of the book is intentionally simple. Each chapter represents a question. The questions in this book are the same questions often asked at my parent presentations. I hope the questions reflect many of the same interests and concerns you have. Some questions will shock you and some may sound unbelievable, I assure you someone asked it. I'd rather express that I have responses and not answers to questions. There is such finality to the term answer, like this is it, end of story.

This book is a collection of my responses, perspectives and insights and I encourage you to read with a curious and open mind.

Many parents and school administrators encouraged me to put my answers down on paper. I have enjoyed answering these questions because I have always felt the "live" presentation format limited my time and ability to share more research. I also felt I edited answers to be politically correct and not offend parents or put the school in an awkward position.

This book serves as "part soapbox" for me. I have spent months answering some questions, rewriting and adding research references, and minutes on others. I imagine you will disagree with some of my responses, and others will validate what you already know and feel.

Ultimately, I hope that the answers spark a dialogue in your family that makes a positive difference for you and your children.

One way to read this book is to skip to those questions that interest you. However, I would encourage you to read them all. Some of my responses will support your current behavior and stimulate your thinking in other areas. One thing is certain; there is no easy or singular path to parenting teens. It is a never ending flux of compromises, fear regulation, and personal exploration of your own childhood wounds, and faith.

Parenting teens will inevitably reveal your own wounds from childhood and we all have them. In some ways, I think the job of a parent is to recognize your own childhood wounds and not pass them on to your own children. Whenever I get into this area during a parent presentation, I will see someone crying in my audience. We are all wounded. It's a question of whether you are going to parent from those wounds or heal them.

We live in a fast paced culture where speed and efficiency is worshipped. Speed and efficiency may be useful and appropriate for getting tasks done, but children are not tasks. In matters of the heart, speed is an obstacle to reflection and wisdom.

My answers are direct and simple and meant to cause reflection that reveals wisdom. I would like to point out that simple answers to complex problems can be seductive. By seductive I mean that a "good looking sound bite" in print or spoken in a media interview may sound good but does it really do the job of getting to the heart of the matter. Underage drinking and other drug use is a complex social problem. Anyone who tells you different is ignorant or completely out of touch with the issue.

My suggestions and insights should be part of your ongoing search for solutions and are certainly not a panacea to them. I hope you are surrounded by wise and supportive friends and family who speak candidly when it is called for.

Draw upon their strength as you attempt to raise your children free of harmful drinking and other drug use.

I have seen firsthand the destructive power of addiction in families. I am deeply committed to helping you avoid the pain I have gone through and the enormous pain I put my family through especially. The fact that I am here to write this book is a testament to my family's and friend's love and support for me.

I hope you enjoy this book and find helpful content in it.

DEFINING TERMS

One of the controversies affecting the field of prevention is the inability of practitioners, researchers, and educators to agree on a precise definition of what prevention is. The word "prevention" has different meanings to different people. The guy sitting next to me on a flight who asks what I do for a living thinks I get kids off of drugs—a noble goal, however not prevention, but intervention and treatment. Another person thinks about the D.A.R.E (Drug Awareness Resistance Education) program—a nationally recognized anti-drug program aimed primarily at elementary and middle school aged children—yet another person thinks about immunization shots or medical related issues. At the time of this writing, I lost track of the number of definitions I have read about what prevention means. It seems as if each researcher or program establishes a definition of prevention to best suit their own goals.

For the purposes of this book I use the word prevention as a descriptor of any program, attitude, behavior, activity or approach that attempts to support and encourage those students choosing not to drink, and/or aims to reduce the negative impact of drinking and other drug use by teenagers, and/or aims to reduce the frequency and amount of drinking by teens.

You will notice that I say, "alcohol and other drugs" not "alcohol and drugs." This particular phrasing itself is a controversy. The former expression is often seen as an attempt to stigmatize alcohol by associating it with the likes of cocaine and heroine. Alcohol is a drug and the use by adolescents should be taken seriously. My wording "alcohol and other drugs" is not a political gesture or an attempt to align myself with a particular philosophy. I'm merely making an attempt to point out that alcohol is a drug, not to demonize alcohol. It is my opinion that alcohol is neither good nor bad. For most people (there are exceptions) alcohol's risk is in how it is used, frequency of use, how much is used and the environment in which it is used.

Binge drinking is a term that most people are familiar with today. In the minds of most people, binge drinking either describes a person on an extended drinking spree lasting more than 24 hours or a person that drinks a lot on a given occasion. The term binge drinking originated from the Harvard School of Public Health during the 1990's.[2][3][4] The current definition of binge drinking is (5) or more drinks for men and (4) or more drinks for women in a single sitting. Now, this is where we run into trouble. What is a single sitting? If a woman has two drinks with dinner and then three glasses of wine over the course of four hours

---

[2] Meilman PW, Cashin JR, McKillip JR, Presley CA. Understanding the three national databases on collegiate alcohol and drug use. *J Am Coll Health*. 1998;46(4):68.

[3] Weschler H. Alcohol and the American college campus: a report from the Harvard School of Public Health. *Change*. 1996;28(4):20 – 25
[4] Weschler H, Dowdall GW, Maenner G, Gledhill – Hoyt J, Lee H. Changes in binge drinking and related problems among American College students between 1993 and 1997. J Am Coll Health. 1998;47(2):57 – 68.

that evening, is she a binge drinker? Or take my dad for instance. He is a big guy. Consuming five or more beers in a single sitting—again how long is that—a round of golf?—is not normally considered a risk for my dad. We could spend all day defining binge drinking. I will use the term *dangerous drinking*[5] in this book. I think we can all agree that dangerous drinking implies drinking beyond your physiological limit with unintended and undesirable consequences. Would dangerous drinking include any amount of alcohol consumed by a minor because they are breaking the law—thus putting them at risk of arrest? I'll let you decide that. How you decide matters; more on that later.

Social Norms (approach), or **social norms marketing** is an environmental strategy gaining ground in health promotion strategies. Researchers discovered that students often exaggerate the frequency and consumption habits of other students regarding alcohol. These exaggerations have been found to be consistent among many higher education institutions and secondary schools. The perceived amounts of drinking and other drug use almost always exceeds actual levels. The social norms approach has been used to counter misperceptions, predominantly as a means to reduce extreme drinking, but it is increasingly applied to other social issues and risky behaviors.

Social drinking/drinker is another term that is used quite often. How best to describe social drinking or a social drinker? I often say social drinking is any drinking that is done is a manner that does not impair social, cognitive or

---

[5] Fern Walter Goodheart, MSPH, CHES, Linda C. Lederman, PhD, Lea P. Stewart, PhD, and Lisa Laitman, MSEd., Binge Drinking: not the word of change. P. 204, article 52, Annual Editions, Drugs, Society, and Behavior.

physical functioning. However, the science that informs the drinking and driving debate suggest that impairment begins on the first drink. Also, all of us know someone whose personality changes after one drink. Maybe they become more relaxed, more social and at ease. Is this still social drinking? Or is alcohol doing something for them that they can't do for themselves? Are you starting to see why this gets a little fuzzy? Our struggle to understand and define these behaviors and attach simple labels eludes many and drives the confusion among adults.

Substance use versus **substance abuse** is another sticky issue. Many people believe that any substance use by an adolescent is abuse because of the illegality. Using the public policy model (breaking the law) the answer would be yes. Neurologically speaking, one could argue abuse and use vary from person to person and amount and duration of the substance use. Where do you stand? These are important questions to think about. Many kids have asked me what is worse for you pot or alcohol? What they are really asking is what is worse for you getting drunk or getting high. My answer is neither; it is like switching seats on the Titanic. However, science supports the position that getting drunk is far worse than getting intoxicated on marijuana. Would you share that with a group of tenth graders?

However, getting high on marijuana causes neurological impairment and a personality change that social drinking does not. New research on adolescent neurological development suggests there is no such thing as a safe amount of alcohol or other drugs in the teenage brain. Is this abuse of marijuana? How about getting stoned, but no unintended or undesirable consequences happened? Use or abuse of marijuana? Talking to teens becomes a process infused with agendas, falsehoods, and socially constructed taboos.

The illegality of substances has very little to do with addictiveness, think of alcohol and tobacco-compounding the complexity of prevention work with teens. Addiction Specialist Stanton Peele describes addiction as a consequence of involvement with absorbing experiences that provide essential emotional satisfactions but that detract from people's ability to cope with their lives.

How we define terms or understand these controversies matters. It shapes your approach as a practitioner, informs your belief system as an administrator shaping school policy, and it affects the decisions you make as a parent. It is useful to think about how you may have defined these terms previously and give some thought to how you feel about them now. I suggest you sit down with your spouse or partner and discuss these terms and clear up any areas of conflict.

One goal of this book is to make you more comfortable speaking with the children in your life about alcohol and other drug issues. If you and your spouse/partner are on separate pages regarding these issues, that will be picked up by your kids. You are and will be for a long time the primary influence in your child's life. Most of the research on adolescent drinking and other drug use shows that parents have the most influence on a teen's decision to drink and use other drugs. We must understand how we feel about these terms to be better communicators.

The fact that you picked up this book tells me you are up to the challenge! Millions of teens make it through the teen years and into adulthood free of addiction and any harms caused by drinking or other drug use. It is possible and a reasonable expectation as a parent that your teen maintain a drug-free lifestyle. I do not want you to assume otherwise or be peer pressured by other parents to let down your guard. If problems arise, deal with them straight on and honestly. Involve the proper professionals to guide you through the turbulent time. But always, always, maintain faith and strength in pursuing a no-use message in your home throughout the teen years.

Blessings.

CHAPTER 1

I'm not very knowledgeable about drugs. How could I tell if my child is using drugs?

This is a difficult question because many of the characteristics of being an adolescent resemble drug use. If I were to say, "Look for abrupt changes in mood, appetite or social affiliations," most of you would run screaming home assuming your kids were on drugs. Adolescents, unlike most adults, often are able to disguise the physical damage and attributes associated with substance abuse because they are young and resilient. Adolescents tend to bounce back faster from a night of drinking than adults.

The mere fact you asked the question is a healthy sign that you are making room for the idea that your child could be using drugs, including alcohol. As long as your feeling does not grow into paranoid intrusiveness, then I think it is a healthy dose of realism on your part. I have met too many parents who say, "I know my daughter and she would never do drugs." Sure, and any day now we are going to find Weapons of Mass Destruction.

My work with independent school adolescents has made me believe that they may be more at risk than their public school counterparts. I met a young lady name Loren at a school in Connecticut.

She approached me after class and said, "I smoke pot (long pause) and I don't think it's working out." Curious I asked, "What do you mean by not working out?" "Well, my grades are fine, athletics are going well, my teachers like me, and my parents and I get along well too, but…" "But what?" I asked. "Smoking weed is the only think that makes me happy." Loren, like many independent school students I meet is an intelligent and gifted student. In many ways, her gifts disguise her developing emotional and psychological reliance on marijuana. I am sure many of the adults in Loren's life would be surprised to learn about her relationship with marijuana, especially her parents.

Loren is a good example of how parents can be surprised by the discovery of substance in their kids. However, I feel there are always clues if the parent *wants* to look.

I have read behavioral checklists that stretch for miles about the physical and emotional symptoms that indicate alcohol and other drug use. I can save you a lot of time by simply stating what I consider to be the most salient signal—your intuition. If your intuition is telling you something is wrong, then listen to it.

Far too often, whether it is in a school setting or family, when it is discovered that a child is using alcohol or other drugs, inevitably someone will say, "I felt that something was not quite right." With your intuitive voice as your guide, here are some additional signs to look for:

- An over-developed sense of privacy
- An avoidance of high commitment activities (school and family)

- An abnormal clash with family values, rituals and beliefs beyond the normal (you define normal based on previous behavior)
- A slide in school performance like academics or not participating in a sport they had in the past—with little reason for it.
- Preoccupation with drug related lifestyle (music/clothing/literature/speech/posters/paraphernalia)

It is important to realize that these signs can be indicators of many other non-drug related issues. You may want to keep this in mind if you decide to speak to your child regarding the changes you have seen in them. Absolutely avoid using accusatory and judgmental language. Initially, your concerns should be about "observable" behavior. I would not speculate as it will only encourage debate and defensiveness.

The signs may be normal adolescent moodiness, the emergence of a learning disability, social problems at school, or just a bad hair day. I do want to emphasize my personal belief that if you have concerns about what you see in your child's life, you have the right and responsibility to speak up and express those concerns. If the issue is drug use, then you may be the only one to express concern. It will not be her pot-smoking friends.

Sometimes, just by pointing out what you are seeing can influence your child to make better decisions. Bringing what your child thought as disguised behavior into the light of day can be a form of intervention. The cynic reading this will say, "Yeah, but then the kids will just get better at hiding it." True, that could happen. But not saying anything will not change anything either.

Either way, you must express concern. I met a young man who was a sophomore at the time. He told me that he smoked pot on and off throughout ninth grade. He said he stopped recently and I asked him why. "My parents made it such a hassle," he said. They were always up when I came home, consistently checked on my whereabouts, and were involved in my school life. I was putting so much energy into not getting caught smoking pot I realized it wasn't worth it anymore." Nice job mom and dad!

If your adolescent does not offer a reasonable explanation for these mood or behavioral changes, you may want to become more vigilant about their coming and goings. Do not be afraid to consult with the school counselor, get feedback from your child's teachers, or other professionals. You don't have to say, "Hey, I think my kid is smoking pot!" But you could start gathering more information to inform your growing concern and guide your next step.

It is important to remember that when an adolescent's drug use is recognized by the adult community, it usually has been going on for some time. Discovering paraphernalia in their room, a beer bottle cap in the back seat of your car after they borrowed it or the smell of tobacco or marijuana on their coat is not likely to be the first time—as many adolescents will claim and too many adults are willing to believe. Hopeful thinking like, "Maybe this is the first time?" is usually just that—hopeful thinking. Hopeful thinking deepens the problem.

Address the issue assertively and openly. All drug use and the potential emergence of a dependency grows fast and furious in the cover of darkness and denial. Do not offer the fertilizer of embarrassment and shame.

CHAPTER 2

If I discover my child is using drugs, what do I do?

Unlike adults, it is difficult to assess the severity of drug use with adolescents. Since an adolescent's use of alcohol is illegal, many people consider any use to be abuse. Yet, there are distinct differences between adult and adolescent chemical use. For example, an adult who drinks in the morning to stave off withdrawal symptoms or to face the day would be considered chemically dependent. Yet, a child using before school may not be an indicator of drug dependence. It may simply be a cool thing to do, a response to a dare, or extremely bad judgment as influenced by peers. However, my professional experience tells me that a teen drinking or using other drugs before or during school is a red flag of concern. An adult hiding their alcohol or other drug use is a sure sign of dependence, but for adolescents it is a common behavior. Parents who discover their child has been using drugs or alcohol should consider having an assessment conducted by a trained substance abuse counselor. I strongly recommend not using the family pediatrician for this assessment, unless your pediatrician has psychiatric and chemical dependency training as well.

The trained counselor will be able to recognize signs of denial and be better prepared to discuss treatment options with parents if necessary. I will add a bit of caution here:

Should the counselor tell you that he or she thinks that the problem has not progressed to dependency, this does not mean the teen is out of the woods. Counselors are trained professionals, not mind readers. They can only work with what they are told. If counseling is suggested for the adolescent, I encourage parents to attend counseling sessions as well. A child using alcohol and/or other drugs is always a family issue. Unless everyone is willing to look at the family dynamics that may be creating, enabling, and influencing the drug use, the behavior will only be superficially treated and is likely to pop up again and again.

In a recent study comparing traditional adolescent substance abuse treatment options such as individual and group therapy with family-centered therapy, also known as multi-systemic therapy (MST), the traditional approaches of individual and group therapy showed significantly poorer results. In other words, don't dump your kids off at the rehab or therapy session and say, "fix'em!"

Adolescents can and do heal when the family is included in the intervention, treatment and after-care support.

Very rarely, and never in my professional experience working with adolescents in a treatment setting, does an adolescent who is experiencing chemical dependency or mental health issues heal without the intervention and support of the adults in their life.

Adolescent substance abuse occurs within a system of enablers—peers, school, parents, and community enablers like police—and it takes a system to break a system.

Maintaining privacy is a concern for many parents when addressing their child's substance use. However, I would encourage parents to share part or all of the substance abuse assessment with the school. Mental health counselors and other health related school personnel could be supportive allies in a student's recovery and reintegration into the community after a student has experienced inpatient or outpatient care.

Adolescent substance abuse is a systemic problem, meaning, a child's use of drugs occurs in several domains; their school, their community, their family, and their peer group. To intervene effectively, the more that the healthy domains are working together in collaboration, the more effective the intervention will be.

I suggest schools adopt an "assess and meet" approach following any substance related policy violation by a student. For example, it is wise to having a meeting between the parents, student, school representative (Advisor) and therapist to chart out a course of treatment and to talk about "what next" options should the teen slip back into old patterns.

Establishing a "what next" position avoids any confusion as to what will happen if the teen relapses back into drug using behavior. It sets a tone and a course of action for stepping up treatment when appropriate and as needed.

Adopting the approach, "Let's try this and see what happens" is not a good plan. It is better to be prepared for relapse behavior than ignore the possibility it could occur.

It is difficult for most parents and even schools to regard an adolescent getting caught by the school as an opportunity, but it is. Consider that most adolescents who get harmfully involved in substances are using two years before the adult community catches wind of it.

A violation often means that the adolescent is getting careless and is an opportunity to provide an early intervention in the form of counseling and assessment.

Understandably, knowledge that your son or daughter is involved in substance use is frightening. It can be unnerving. With proper assessment, assertive action, and a willingness on the part of the parents to explore the family dynamics that may be supporting and enabling the use, families can heal and emerge stronger from the experience.

Recommended reading

Kuhn, C., (1996). *Buzzed*. MN: Hazeldon Publishing, Inc.

CHAPTER 3

I have one son in the fifth grade and I can already see how intense the peer pressure is getting for him. How can I support him to not give in to it and make decisions for himself?

I think peer pressure is one of those scary issues that parents with children in the elementary and middle school think about a lot. I believe that peer pressure is one of the most misunderstood themes in ATOD (Alcohol, Tobacco & Other Drugs) education. Bring up the word peer pressure with a group of teenagers and you will hear an audible groan "here we go again." Or, they will say, "There's no such thing!" They are partially right. Peer pressure is not what most adults think it is.

It is rare for kids to overtly try to cajole and threaten others to drink and use other drugs. From a very early age, kids begin to hear the message that looming somewhere in the shadows—on the way home from school—exists this nefarious group of people hell bent on getting them to use drugs through any means necessary. For the most part, this image is more "Hollywood" than real life. I have worked in some urban school environments and peer pressure can be more explicit around using substances. However, for the sake of your questions, peer pressure is subtle and more intra-psychic than most people understand.

In a recent study done by the Center of Addiction and Substance Abuse at Columbia University, a large percentage of kids said they got their alcohol at friends' homes or through another adult. When I smoked pot in high school, I got most of my weed through my best friend or his older brother. I bought most of my alcohol from my older brothers and initially tried cocaine with my cousin. Drug use and people that sell drugs do not come in "easy to recognize and avoid" packages. Peer pressure usually comes from the people close(est) to the adolescent: People they trust and feel comfortable with.

Unfortunately, most kids' first experience with drinking is with their parents! How many times have you been at a family event and someone thought it was cute that little Andy was sipping his dad's beer!

We do a disservice to kids by perpetuating this myth of strangers with bad intent. We cannot discount the effect that group dynamics have on decision-making. My father used to say, "If your friends jump off a bridge, would you?" Well, the answer may well be, "probably." Good decision-making in the face of peer pressure is about having a strong sense of self-worth and a trust in your own decision-making.

Parents play a key role in nurturing this belief in their children and guiding their children in clarifying their own beliefs. Barbara Vaccarr, Ph. D, a psychologist and professor at Lesley University suggests that parents ask themselves the following questions when thinking about their children and peer pressure:

> ➢ "How did I deal with peer pressure when I was younger?"

> "What fears do I have about my child being a victim of peer pressure?"

> "How would I want my child to deal with peer pressure?

Vaccarr suggests that children who are able to resist social pressure have an innate sense of being trustworthy; this belief is given to them and reinforced by their parents.

Decision-making is a critical skill for adolescents to develop. Oftentimes parents become too focused on their children reaching the right answer (a.k.a the parents' answer) as opposed to helping them develop a sound *process* of reaching answers. The right decision is subjective and those parents with teenagers will testify to this. We can avoid debates and confrontations that usually arise when we want our children to choose our answer by supporting them in developing the skills of good decision-making and then allowing them to practice making their own decisions.

Early practice in making decisions in easier and more mundane scenarios such as what to wear or read or watch on TV as younger children makes for better decision-making skills as scenarios get tougher in the teen years. The sooner independent decision-making is encouraged, the better for the child in the years when peer pressure becomes a bigger issue.

Also, it is important not to demonize your child's peer group as you seek to understand the influence of close peers on your son and daughter. Overall, peer groups provide more good influences than bad. They provide a sense of belonging, connection, sameness, and a place where the intimacy of friendship can be rehearsed safely. Your teen is being vulnerable with someone that may once have been you but in middle and high school whom they confide in changes. Why not make an effort to get to know your child's closest peers as one means of staying engaged with your child?

Maybe you have heard your teenager explain that an adult was either awesome or an idiot. Teenagers typically apply this same style of thinking in extremes to decision-making when they narrow their options down to *this* or *that*. For example, if I go to the party, I'll have to drink, or if I don't go, everyone will think I'm a loser. Adults can help adolescents explore their options in social situations and show that there is a full spectrum between the extremes.

A good place for parents to start is to understand that boys and girls are under different kinds of peer pressure. Our culture puts heavy emphasis on drinking and masculinity. Boys have a cultural expectation to drink, to define and express their masculinity with alcohol. One young man in 9th grade said to me during class, "When I drink with my friends, I feel big." During another discussion with eighth graders in Philadelphia, I asked, "Would it be easier for a boy or a girl to be alcohol and drug free in high school?" Without hesitation, all of them agreed that it would be easier for a girl. "Why?", I asked. One girl exclaimed, "You just kind of imagine a guy walking around a party with a six-pack of beer in his hand."

The images of masculinity and the connection with alcohol are cumulative for young men. It is the confluence of cognition—the ability to think about themselves—and the emergence of puberty that creates a sort of psychological disequilibrium. This disequilibrium is resolved by grasping for grounding images and behaviors that validate their emerging selves—and sometimes these behaviors become self-sabotaging and potentially destructive.

American culture is in dire need of creating passages—long lost in Western cultures—for both boys and girls to pass through "safely" to mark their development.

In middle school, many Alcohol, Tobacco and Other Drug (ATOD) education programs oversimplify the issue of peer pressure by offering trite expressions like "Just Say No," or scripted responses that most kids recognize as shallow and misguided. There is not enough dialogue nor is it a safe environment for kids to open up and discuss what is really going on among them and their peers. In many ways, family systems and parenting style can be the culprit for creating kids who are more susceptible to negative peer pressure.

Jane Bluestein, President of Educational Resource Center, talks about the conditional love parents attach to desired behaviors as fertile ground for weakness under peer pressure to take root. Children that are raised with the belief that the way to get accepted is to do what they are told will be more susceptible to peer pressure. If acceptance is contingent upon meeting other people's expectations, then this is a set up for how they may behave in the future. What is caving in to peer pressure but a child's inability to trust themselves and their own thoughts and impulses? Imagine a child having a strong enough sense of self or self-concept to realize that, "No matter what the outcome of my decision, I am still a good person."

These messages and images and the core values associated with them start in the home long before a child has to face the challenge of turning down offers of alcohol and other drug use. How then does the societal paradigm of providing students with scripted answers serve as a useful tool against peer pressure? It provides a feel good and easy answer to a complicated problem. We do kids a disservice when we continue to teach them strategies for dealing with peer pressure that ultimately fail.

This failure only compounds the sense of disempowerment and hopelessness that children feel in the powerful social climate of their peers. It takes more effort to develop a leader than a follower and the sooner we promote self-leadership in our children, the stronger they are in difficult situations on their own or in their peer groups.

Children will have a greater likelihood of making good decisions if they know where the boundaries are—the line in the sand, so to speak. Mom and dad are responsible for placing that line and backing it up with consequences when the line is crossed. How do we help our kids navigate peer pressure? As parents and early mentors, we need to send clear messages about expectations around the use of alcohol and other drugs and clear and enforceable consequences when violating those expectations.

Parents need to work at supporting the "process" of decision-making so kids begin to trust their own decisions.

My work with students has taught me many lessons, but the one thing I have learned is that parents are the number one cited reasons for kids saying no to drinking and other drug use. The kids who say no fear the parental disappointment it may cause and value the trust their parents grant them. Parents who acknowledge this attitude in their children and use a positive and constructive parenting style will have greater success equipping their children with real-life tools to deal with peer pressure that is potentially harmful.

In my experience, the most common appearance of alcohol and other drugs is through the existing peer group, not the emergence of a new set of deviant peers. Your son's friends change, he begins to initiate new behaviors, and thus he acquires new friends based on these new behaviors. And this is how the cycle goes throughout middle school and high school. This dramatically changes the equilibrium of the peer group creating a tension which I define as peer pressure.

How your son or daughter navigates these new alliances and their own sense of belonging and disconnection is what is challenging. As they change so should you in how you relate, react and respond. The important point here is stay engaged or get engaged if you are not. Science has informed us that certain protective factors can trump risk factors.

For instance, parents that are actively involved in their children's lives, who know their friends, call ahead to "trust but verify" (what I call the CSI: Home Method), can trump the risk factor of drug using peers.

When I ask students who don't drink or use other drugs why they don't use, I often hear, "It's too much of a hassle—sooner or later I'd get caught and that would ruin everything." The kids who have their parents' trust are saying they want to keep it.

The tendency for parents to connect their peace of mind with their children's choices, achievements or appearance leaves children continually vulnerable to all sorts of things over which they have limited control. (according to Jane Bluestein)

The problem is not peer pressure or social groups trying to cajole kids into drinking or drug use, it is that kids are not connected enough to specific relationships that are growth fostering (Miller and Stiver). In other words, who we associate with matters a great deal and it pays off to be an actively engaged parent throughout the school years.

- Peer pressure is usually not a group of strangers trying to cajole and deceive your child into drinking or using other drugs
- Research confirms that adolescents who drink get their alcohol primarily from adults: a friend's home, older siblings, approaching an adult outside a liquor store, or an older friend.
- Clear, consistent, and enforced boundaries and consequences are helpful to children resisting peer pressure.

Recommended reading

Bluestein, J., (1993). *Parents, teens, and boundaries: how to draw the line.* Deerfield Beach, FL: Health Communications Inc.

Smith, L., & Elliott, C., (2001). *Hollow kids: recapturing the soul of a generation lost to the self-esteem myth.* New York: Random House

CHAPTER 4

My son came home the other day and asked me if I ever did drugs!

I have heard this question at almost every parent meeting I have ever done. It is a tough one and parents struggle with the notion that if they tell their kids that they did drugs, then it gives them permission to do the same. I have never met a student who told me that their reasons for smoking pot were because mom and dad did when they were young.

This question is tricky because it taps into our own childhood memories which may be associated with feelings of guilt or shame and regret.

To help our children though we need to share our wisdom gained from our own experiences: But where details are concerned, be discerning as to how much you choose to include.

I was at an airport years ago waiting for a delayed flight—I do that a lot—and I started a conversation with a woman sitting next to me. After finding out what I do, she asked, "What do I tell my own kids about my history with drinking or drug use?" I gave my answer that I usually give, she nodded with apparent interest. I asked, "What do you think?" "I disagree", she said. "I think you should be totally honest. "Why do you feel that way?" I then asked. She responded, "I grew in house full of lies. I promised myself I would be honest with my kids so they would never suffer the pain of not knowing what is real."

What happened to us as children matters when we become adults and parents for better or for worse.

Most kids appreciate the candor parents can offer in this situation; instead of running from this conversation, look at it as an opportunity to have an open dialogue. This is a loaded question which has surfaced for a reason. Let me make an important point here; if you did not do "**anything**" when you were younger—then the answer is simple. It TOO is a valuable experience to share. Share with your child the reasons why chose not to take the risks. A large percentage of youths do not use alcohol and other drugs. Hopefully, your child is one of those kids and wants to feel supported and may be wondering whether they are normal.

Depending on the age of your child, I believe your answer should reflect an age appropriate response. Consider the factors that surround the conversation like tone and situation. Research does not support one particular approach over another. The question can be handled in a variety of ways. I would recommend parents stay within their comfort zone. Be sure to listen carefully to the verbal and non-verbal clues your child may send you during the conversation. Be thoughtful in your answers. Do not rush thoughts if you are still mulling them over.

Space and silence between answers can be useful in adding depth and meaning to the conversation. If you are unsure of your child's thoughts, ask for feedback—"How do you feel about what I'm saying?"

What follows are a few more ideas. As a parent you should keep the following questions in mind:

- ➤ What is my son really asking?
- ➤ Why is my daughter asking this question?
- ➤ What does my son already know?
- ➤ How much information does my daughter need?

Often at the end of these fact finding questions, parents find that the child has lost interest in whether or not "mom" did drugs and is more interested in why people try drugs—a behavior they are learning has dire consequences.

Parents should also realize that pausing, taking a moment and allowing silence to infuse the conversation often gives the child and the parent a moment to think about their responses and attach deeper meaning to what has been said or will be said. It is okay for parents to say, "I do not know" or "You know I will have to think about that and get back to you."

The Freedom Institute located in New York City provides the following series of scripted responses. These may be helpful for some parents.

Elementary:

> **Daughter:** "Mom did you use drugs when you were a kid?"
> **Mother:** "It sounds like you are studying drugs/health in school?"
> **Daughter:** "Yeah, my teacher Ms. Adler said drugs were bad and a lot of people do drugs"

> **Mother**: "When you say the word "drug" what kinds of things come to mind? Because there are good drugs and bad drugs."
> **Daughter**: "I don't know I guess…" "I suppose she meant bad drugs"
> **Mother**: "When you say bad drugs, can you be specific?"

Middle School:

I would encourage parents to initially follow the same line of dialogue as with the elementary child. Many parents will discover however that their child may still return to the question, "Mom, did you try drugs?" Let's pick up the conversation from there:

> **Son**: "Dad, did you try drugs?"
> **Father**: "Wow, it sounds as if you're learning about drugs in school?"
> **Son**: "Well, just about alcohol and drugs, the teacher said a lot of people your age used drugs when they were young."
> **Father**: "I don't know what your teacher meant to say, but I can tell you about those times. Would you like me to?" (Give the child the choice. Some will not want to pursue the topic any further, others will)
> **Son**: "Sure."
> **Father**: "Many people my age who were young adults back then tried marijuana. We mostly called it pot. But we didn't know as much about it as we do now. It was the same with cigarettes. We didn't think smoking was very harmful either. So do you still want to know if I smoked marijuana? Think about your answer. How would you feel if I said yes?

Son: "I'll have to think about it. Well, yes and no. Yes, because you always said it's important to be honest. No, because I'm not sure what I'll think about you. If you say no, you'll just be a regular parent. If you say yes, I don't know—it may be kind of weird."
Father: "You're exactly right. That's why I want you to think about it. But remember, whatever you decide is okay, and whatever my answer is, we can talk more about it.

If you decide to tell your child that you did "try" drugs, you may want to follow the following steps outlined below.

Upper School:

> ➤ Be honest. Adolescents can tell when adults are being evasive.

> ➤ Recognize that many people in your generation started using alcohol or other drugs much later in their teens, probably in college. There is a significant reduction of risk associated with alcohol and other drug used at later ages. Make your children aware of the dangers of using chemicals during adolescence and tell them the risks associated with starting at an early age.

> ➤ Listen, listen, and listen some more! Parents often ask, "How can I get my son to talk with me?" I urge them to listen more and speak less. In addition, my former business partner Brenda always made this important point; adults always expect kids to get out of their comfort zone and discuss personal issues.

Yet, parents rarely reciprocate. In order for trust to be built and conversations to go deeper, each person needs to be willing to take some risks.

- If you did "use", share the consequences of your use. Tell them what you learned from the experience. If there weren't any consequences, I'm sure you can think of other people you know whose relationship with substance use was not a successful one. Don't exaggerate or lie. Your son or daughter will find out the truth from someone and not trust you again for accurate information. If you don't know the answer to something concerning drugs, turn it into a project by saying, "I don't know, but would like to, let's find out together."

- Avoid lecturing and moralizing. View the conversation as ongoing, not a one-stop fix where everything has to be said. When I work with kids in schools, they usually take the entire four days with me to get to that one question that is foremost in their minds. They are usually spending their initial time evaluating whether I'm safe and trustworthy. Trust takes time to build and but a moment to break. Remember that with your kids.

No other question in all my years of doing this work has changed as much as this one. I do not believe in total honesty, especially with younger children. I like to call this "selective editing." I think younger children build their ideas of a safe world around the consistency and image of mom and dad. The news of mom being a pot smoker may be honest, but very difficult for an adolescent to understand or accept. In most cases, when younger children (K-6) have asked this question of me, I have found that their real curiosity lies elsewhere.

I was giving a presentation to a large group of six graders in Brooklyn when during the question and answer session a young man asked, "Mr. Wolfsberg, did you ever do drugs?" I paused for a moment and said, "Wow, that's a big question." I often pause when answering questions of younger students to allow time for their words to catch up with their thinking.

To his credit he just stared me down waiting for an answer. I continued, "I remember thinking a lot about that when I was your age. Who did drugs, why they did them; I imagine you're thinking a lot about that during a presentation like this?" The young man jumped in excitedly, "Yeah, exactly, why would a person do drugs when they know it's bad for them?"

In most cases, I do not believe that young children are interested in whether we did drugs or not. But they are looking for an adult to recognize and connect to the greater question behind their question, "Do you know how I feel?"

I think dad's have to be especially careful when they share their stories of "passage." as their son's approach adolescence In an attempt to bond, a father can romanticize the first and subsequent times getting drunk with buddies. This kind of storytelling as I think of it, is not helpful. Some selective editing may be helpful until your child has reached an age of lesser risk.

Review

- What is really being asked when they ask, "Mom, did you ever smoke pot?"
- It is okay to decide that you are uncomfortable with the answering the question.
- It is less about who you were back then, and more important to connect with your current responsibility as a parent now.
- For younger children, use selective editing and build in reflection time.

CHAPTER 5

If I suspect my child is using drugs, is it alright for me to snoop in her room?

There is a big difference between snooping and exploring a concern. I think it is important to respect and honor your child's privacy. If you expect them to respect yours, then they deserve the same. I do not agree with "my house my rules" mentality that often justifies inappropriate boundary intrusions.

Good communication will allow you to gain most of the information you need to address your concerns. The need to snoop usually means there is a disconnect between effective communication and trust in the home.

There are limits to my belief of course. I think if your daughter has a history of suicide, or if there is a pattern of behavior that indicates violence or substance use, then safety concerns trump honoring privacy.

If you have concrete observable concerns or some proof such as "found a marijuana pipe while doing her laundry" then breaking privacy feels appropriate to me. Without these elements, I feel the violations can have the opposite of the desired effect.

Growing up my dad was and still is in some ways a very intrusive man. To his credit he has learned to be more aware of boundaries and honor them. I remember in high school getting my own post office box in order to get my mail so that dad would not read it. He always claimed, "I thought it was mine." One Saturday, I bumped into my two brothers and my mother at the post office—all of us furtively checking our own post office boxes.

A parent who violates boundaries without cause can create a scenario where alcohol and other drug use becomes the "private ownership" of the adolescent. I remember thinking in high school when drinking, "This is mine." I felt my dad could not and would not own or know about this. It worked.

Adolescents should gain and grow in the area of privacy and ownership. Without it, the possibility of two extremes develops. One extreme is they cannot make any decision independently or the other is they make all the wrong decisions very independently in spite!

Review

> ➢ Boundary intrusions are often about control. Be honest with yourself when deciding whether to enter your child's room, check their pockets, or search their car. Is this behavior short-cutting the need for better communication?
> ➢ Respect their privacy if you expect them to respect yours.
> ➢ Inspecting a room, looking through a backpack, or checking the pockets of discarded clothing should have justified reasons such as a history of behavioral problems with clear and present suspicious ions.

Recommended reading

Sells, S., (2001). *Parenting your out-of-control teenager: 7 steps to reestablish authority & reclaim love.* New York: NY, St. Martin's Press

CHAPTER 6

I want my son to trust me—yet what should I do when he tells me that a friend of his drinks and uses other drugs? I know this kid and his parents, but I don't want to break my son's trust.

Whenever I hear this question, it reminds of a question almost all students ask me the first day of a seminar, "Is what we say to you confidential?" My answer is "It depends." If your son is telling you something that obviously constitutes an immediate danger to someone like suicide or homicidal feelings, then all bets are off.

I do think there are some non-negotiable issues. I remember facilitating a parent-student evening at a school in Virginia when this issue came up. Parent and students were mixed into groups with a list of discussion questions. One father addressed the question of trust by saying, "Once you break their (children) trust, forget about them every talking with you again." There was a long pause, then an eighth grade boy spoke up, "That's not true, I talk with my dad all the time about stuff, but he's my dad and sometimes dads got to do dad stuff, like... tell it like it is." My belief is most kids know where the line is that separates issues of concern and crisis.

I think it is natural to struggle with this question. I've struggled with answering it for years. I think I finally understand why I struggle with it. There is really no simple answer. The answer lies within the relationship of the individuals involved. For instance, one father may have an honest relationship with another father whose kids know each other. He may be in the position to tell his friend, "Hey, my son shared some information regarding your son's drug use. He shared it in confidence, and I need you to help me out on this one. I would take a closer look at where and what your son is up too. I'm working things out with my son, but I think we need to work together to put a stop to this." It all depends on who are the people involved and if these people can work together honestly.

Your child has given you a piece of disturbing information, and now the question is what to do with it. As a parent you turn it around in your head and say, "Would I want to know?" Most parents say they want to know, but the stories of parents who've made the phone call of concern to the other parent only to be met with a curt and defensive retort are endless. If you tell the other parent, your son or daughter will never trust you again you think. What are the alternatives?

First, I don't think adolescents feel the dagger of betrayal as deeply as the feeling that they weren't involved, consulted, or listened to about a solution.

What makes this question difficult to answer is that it requires a process oriented solution—meaning there are no quick fixes. Here in the United States we are plagued by "McParenting." Most parents want quick, one size fits all, and easy-to-apply solutions to their family communication problems. Questions like the one we are addressing here require high trust levels between individuals and are process oriented.

The first step may very well be telling your daughter, "Listen, I've been thinking about what you told me the other day and I'm really worried about your friend. I don't want to overreact, but can we talk more about what's going on with this friend?"

In my experience, adolescents get less anxious when they feel that you are not going to run off and do something reactionary. Time and time again, I hear students tell me, "I don't tell my parents stuff because they just blow up." Depending on the age of your son—I'll assume an upper school level for this vignette—you may have to take off your parent hat and put on your consultant hat.

Ask questions, "Does the school have a Student Assistance Team where we can make a referral, possibly anonymously?" You could add, "I'd really feel better if we took some positive action." Now is a good time to discuss trust again. You've built trust by listening and consulting on a solution. You've also enhanced your son's decision-making skills by brainstorming and listening carefully to what he had to say—not randomly dismissing his ideas. Instead of saying, "I don't want you to hang around with that kid anymore!" You may try:

> ➤ "I trust you enough to maintain this friendship, but I'm still uncomfortable with you hanging around someone who is drinking and using other drugs."

> ➤ "What do you see as the risks in continuing this relationship?"

> "Can we talk about some alternatives so I can get more comfortable? I'm concerned that his drinking will put you in a risky situation like drinking and driving. Can we talk about that?"

Adolescents take their relationships seriously. They take their role in their friendships seriously too. When an adolescent decides to share with an adult a troubling experience with a friend, it is important to remember it is their *experience*. For girls, self-esteem is linked to how they build, maintain and nurture their friendships. These experiences with friends are growth-fostering experiences that are the foundation of their emerging selves.[6]

Trust is only present when a healthy relationship exists between people. Within that relationship, each person has to realize that the other will not act without regard for the other. If you've built trust over the years, then your child will trust you to do the right thing. It is critical to remember this when talking through sensitive material.

Most kids get uneasy about giving adults information because they are not sure how that information is going to be used. It is important that your child know how and when you are going to use the information he or she shared. Parents need to remember that they are the parent, the grown up, and should be prepared to take responsibility for

---

[6] Carol Gilligan is widely known for her work on female adolescent development. Her concept of "ethic of care" is critical when recognizing how young women perceive relationships. My thoughts have been further developed by the work of Jean Baker Miller and Irene Stiver in such books as the Healing Connection (1997) and Women's Growth in Connection: Writings from the Stone Center (1991)

sharing information with others even if it means not being liked for a time by their own son or daughter.

Recommended reading

Gilligan, C., (1984). *In a different voice.* Cambridge, MA: Harvard University Press.

Miller, J. B., & Stiver, I., (1996). *The healing connection.* Boston, MA: Beacon Press.

CHAPTER 7

Alcoholism runs in our family; when should I tell my kids about it?

Would you talk to your kids about smoking if cancer or heart disease ran in the family? Would you encourage your children to exercise and eat healthy foods if diabetes ran in the family? If your answer is yes, then I would discuss alcoholism.

Alcoholism was recognized as a disease in 1959 by the American Medical Association. Since then, research has suggested a genetic component. Contrary to myth, there is no gene for alcoholism, but the latest research indicates it may be more a confluence of gene types that formulate a risk for certain individuals that is higher in those with a family history of alcoholism.

I will never forget the conversation I had with a teenager I was working with at an inpatient drug treatment center. We were preparing his after-care plan, which would detail where he is going after treatment and what specific activities he was going to do to support his recovery. I asked, "Will you be returning home to mom and dad?" "No, he said, "dad is in treatment in the adult unit." "And mom?" I asked. "She's in the female unit." "Do you have a grandparent that you can live with?" I prodded. "No, my grandmother died of cirrhosis of the liver from drinking and my grandfather is in the elder unit."

This story is not causal and does not necessarily support the idea of genetic risk, but certainly demonstrates the connectedness between nature and nurture when we think of genetic risk.

Alcoholism carries with it moral baggage that still prevents many families from talking about it due to shame and a perceived need for secrecy. At what age should we begin talking with kids about family history? This is a tricky question and has a lot to do with how well you know your child's maturity and developing social life. Ask your school what the health curriculum is and at what point will your son or daughter be discussing alcohol and other drugs. Maybe that would be the right time to open up the discussion about the family's history. Then again, maybe you have an alcoholic relative who is giving you ample opportunities.

There is nothing like a ruined family function to discuss alcoholism in the family. These awkward moments can be turned into excellent teachable moments. Regardless of a family's attempts to hide a family member's alcohol or other drug problem, kids usually are aware it. While younger children may speak out unknowingly out of curiosity, the older siblings may notice and simply say nothing. The bottom line: all these collective experiences color their future behavior where alcohol and drug use are concerned. My suggestion would be to be proactive and talk about what will at first be difficult but could bring healing to a multi-generational family with a history of addictive behaviors.

Here are some guidelines to think about when having a conversation with your children:

- I believe it is important to emphasize the difference between being pre-disposed (high risk) and doomed (destiny).

- I also think it's a wonderful opportunity to express your feelings about alcohol and other drug use and tell them how alcoholism can be **avoided**. Try to stress that alcoholism is a health issue, people get sick and do recover if they receive help. Moralizing the sickness or demonizing alcohol only confuses the real issue.

- Reinforce the idea that you want them to remain abstinent as long as possible to minimize the risk.

- If you drink, discuss the differences between adult drinking and adolescents drinking. This usually can be accomplished by discussing the intent of drinking. Adults with a healthy relationship with alcohol are social drinkers (they drink but not to get drunk) versus adolescent drinking (usually always to excess).

- If you have a daughter, it may be useful to discuss the effects of alcohol that are unique to women. Most alcohol and other drug prevention messages do not recognize gender differences. I think it will be more useful if you tailor your message for your child's gender. Typically speaking, adolescent girls and women tend to get intoxicated and sicker quicker than men. The length of time from the first onset of drinking to dependence is shorter for women than men due to a number of physiological characteristics. In addition to the physiological risks, girls and women have more to worry about when drinking to excess; issues such as sexual assault, unplanned sexual activity, physical assault and date rape.

The bottom line here is don't be scared away from answering this question. Step out of your comfort zone as the parent and tackle the tough material with as much openness, authenticity and transparency as you can. And if you need guidance, most of the schools I work with have talented and knowledgeable counselors on staff willing to role-play a conversation and give you additional tips about handling this very important conversation.

CHAPTER 8

How soon should I begin talking to my kids about alcohol and other drugs?

This is one of those, "It depends on whom you talk too" situations. My partner tells a story of being in a classroom of second graders. She started class by goofing with the kids saying she was from the Federal Chemicals Department and she asked, "What kinds of chemicals do you think we'll discuss today?" The kids responded with, "Fertilizer!"

Prevention programs for substance abuse are in almost every school in the United States. On average, schools provide 14 prevention activities and 90% of public schools provide some information on alcohol, tobacco, drugs, and other risky sexual behavior. Drug Abuse Resistance Education (D.A.R.E) is at the time of this writing in 48% of elementary schools nationwide. Most drug education begins in American schools around the fifth grade with the nationally recognized D.A.R.E program. One of the criticisms of the D.A.R.E program has been that it stimulated curiosity in drugs as opposed to inoculating children against drug use—its intended purpose. In this case, ignorance may be bliss and it may be all that is needed for a time. However, at some point when information, exposure and/or availability arrive, ignorance once a protective factor may now increase the risk factor. Carlo

DiClemente (2003), a specialist in how people change in and out of addictive behaviors explains, "Such approaches may awaken them to the possibilities and make the addictive behavior more salient than it would be in the natural environment (p.71). The trick is to structure and time a prevention program at this precise time—which is difficult!

Most experts will agree that alcohol and drug education has to follow cognitive and emotional development. True, but not all children develop at the same rate. In some fifth grade classes I have had children who knew a lot about alcohol and other drugs while other classmates were very naïve. Unfortunately, my experience with younger children who were knowledgeable about alcohol and other drugs, it was because they were exposed to abusive drinking by the adults in their lives. As one fifth grader put it, "I know a lot about alcohol, my dad gets drunk and my mom and me go to a hotel for a few days."

It is important to know your children and take their emotional temperature from time-to-time to see if they are ready to handle certain themes. I would check with the school about the timing of their alcohol and other drug prevention and perhaps schedule "your talk" around that time to increase the chance of an interesting dialogue.

The most powerful message you send to your children will always be your own behavior.

How is alcohol handled in your home? Is it omnipresent at every family event? Could your children come to the conclusion that adults in the home find it necessary to drink in order to relax or have a good time? Do you model variety in how to recreate and cope with stress and challenges?

Drinking in the home is not a bad thing. However, it is important that parents are aware of the subtle messages they may be sending about the meaning of alcohol in the home.

One mother shared with me a story of driving her seventh grader to school one morning. During conversation on the drive the seventh grader said he noticed the empty bottle of wine in the trash that morning. He said, "Didn't you buy the wine on Monday mom?" The mother was caught off guard and had no idea that her children were that aware of when alcohol comes into the home and when it is gone. Apparently her children are.

Adolescents are very aware of how much and why adults drink. A colleague from years ago told me the story of working with a group of third graders. She asked them, "When do adults drink?" Waiting for the usual "parties" "football games" instead one young lady said, "When they take their coats off." Surprised, my friend asked for further clarification. "Well, at my house, when my daddy answers the door, he always says, "Can I take your coat and get you a drink?"

CHAPTER 9

What are some of the drug trends today?

Alcohol and marijuana is King. I believe it will always be that way due to the value our society places on alcohol use and the passive physical and emotional consequences our culture attaches to marijuana. That aside, trends come and go, but by and large most things aren't new but repackaged. Ecstasy created a lot of buzz when the police and media took notice. I started seeing it long before it hit the U.S in my overseas work. However, Ecstasy isn't new, but a repackaging of a drug that has been around since the 1920's.

There are many web sites out there where parents and educators can get accurate and up-to-date information about the latest drugs. You can start with the National Institute of Drug Abuse and from there be directed to many other science-based web sites devoted to specific drugs like "club drugs" and inhalants. It is always wise to stay informed about the trending drugs and how they are referred to by those using them.

K2 and Spice for example may sound harmless when referred to as incense but in truth they are anything but. It is a parent's responsibility to stay aware of the vernacular their children are using and may be exposed to.

An important aspect of drug trends is called generational forgetting. It is a term attached to the phenomena that when one generation experiences the devastating consequences of one drug, then there is usually a drop in use in the next generation. However, the following generation, having forgotten the consequences of the drug reestablishes a relationship with it and the cycle begins again.

There are also other trends driven by how a drug is used. Heroin had very low levels of use for years due to its intravenous method of use. Then in the late 1980s and early nineties, heroin became so pure it could be snorted up a user's nose with the same intense effects of needle use. This deceptively less threatening method of use opened the door to a whole new group of users scared off by the needle and consequences like HIV and Hepatitis C.

It is important to note that drug use is driven by many factors; social norms, availability and other environmental conditions, social policy, interdiction measures. Social norms have a powerful effect over drug trends. Prescription drug use is escalating and I believe will continue to do so as long as the American culture continues along the lines of self-medicating stressful emotions and experiences. A recent television program by Peter Jennings stated that Americans spent 90 billion more on prescriptions drugs than they did a mere six years ago.

There has been an 800% increase in anti-depressant medication use in the last ten years. Are we really that more depressed? I think these trends require our attention as much as and if not more so than minor swings, although alarming, in illicit drug use.

The trends that are more remarkable may be in our attitudes towards ATOD (Alcohol, Tobacco and Other Drugs).

At the time of this writing a trend that is alarming is the increasing use and abuse of prescription drugs. Although most drug trends are not exclusive to one country, however, I think the use and abuse of prescription drugs is unique to the United States.

CHAPTER 10

What do I do if my child has come home drunk?

Initially, I would assess his/her risk for alcohol poisoning. Does he need to go to the hospital or to bed? Once the safety issue is assessed, assuming you don't kill him yourself, what happens in the morning is very important. Do what you can with your spouse or partner to relieve some of the emotions around the event. Hopefully, long before this incident, you've established clear consequences for such a possible breach in trust. Now should be the time to initiate those consequences. A simple formula to follow may be, 1) Determine the problem behavior—you came home drunk 2) Select fair punishment—should already be established 3) State punishment, 4) Follow through. The hard part really is following through on the consequences. I want to emphasize that the trust between parent and child has been broken. It will and should take time for that trust to be reestablished.

Trust is built upon three pillars: accountability, responsibility, and dependability. These elements need to be reexamined in the light of the specific episode. Love however, is not conditional. It is probably why you are so mad. In addition to expressing your concerns regarding the drinking and initiating the consequences, adolescents are interested in how they can reestablish trust. At some point in the near future, another conversation about how trust will be regained may be useful.

If you want to show that you mean what you say regarding trust and consequences, it will be uncomfortable for a period of time after incidents. Relaxing on a stated consequences potentially sends the message, "I don't fully mean what I say when I say coming home drunk is unacceptable." In short, say what you mean, and mean what you say, and accept that it makes more work for you till lessons are learned and integrated. Children actually appreciate parents who stand their ground and set healthy boundaries.

For many parents, a child coming home drunk or getting a call from the school that their son has committed a substance abuse violation of the school's policy is a startling wake-up call. How parents respond to either of these situations is a moment of truth for the family.

Create time to take a moment, with your spouse or partner, to reflect on why you think this has happened. Is there something within the family system that has contributed to this event? Have you been getting a little too relaxed in your monitoring of your child's social life, his or her comings and goings? Are you giving mixed messages about alcohol? Should some assessment take place to determine severity and extent of the drinking or other drug use?

I think one of the mistakes my father and mother made with me during my adolescent drinking years is that they didn't view my drinking episodes as a health concern to be examined more closely. Adolescent drinking is a furtive activity taking place under the cover and assistance of friends and at times adults. If you have younger children, it may be useful to speak with them about how they are processing the event. Explain how Mom and Dad feel about the use of alcohol and other drugs, and why you have responded the way you have.

There are a number of books available to parents about how to deal with a substance-abusing teenager. One of my favorites is by Dick Schaefer, *Choices and Consequences*. In addition, self-help groups like ALANON and parent support groups are useful places to connect with other parents for support. And finally, if you have a school counselor or school psychologist you trust, they can provide you with support and encouragement.

Recommended reading

Shaefer, D., (1987). *Choices and consequences*. MN: Hazeldon Publishing Inc.

CHAPTER 11

How do I support and encourage my child not to use alcohol and other drugs?

May I suggest and encourage using a prevention oriented approach? Effective prevention programs are based on "models." Models offer a theory of what causes adolescents to drink and use other drugs. Based on these theories, a strategy is adopted by a school to address the risk factors. In the best case scenarios, models and strategies are consciously chosen. However, a model is always at work whether or not it is chosen intentionally or not.

Why is this important? Because parents also have their own ideas of what causes a teen to use alcohol and other drugs. This "model" will drive their decisions and construct their ideas about setting limits and consequences for their teen.

For instance, if a parent is of the belief that only teens with high risk backgrounds like, poverty, low self-esteem, or social alienation are susceptible to chemical dependence, then they set up their children for disaster if their children do not fall into those categories. We know that parents and teens who have the idea that drugs are either soft or hard increase the risks associated with drug use. Students who hold the idea of soft and hard drugs are less likely to use cocaine and heroin (a.k.a. hard drugs) but more likely to use alcohol and marijuana (a.k.a. soft drugs) than those adolescents that do not hold this belief. I think many parents would fall into this category too.

I think what is crucial between parents and teen is a clear expectation that alcohol and other drug use are unacceptable choices during adolescence. This expectation must be set early, communicated often with love, and backed-up with consequences if tested.

In a recent study (2003) conducted by the Center for Alcohol and Substance Abuse (CASA), forty-one percent of parents surveyed said future drug use by *their* children was likely, but only 11 percent of teens gave that response. All too often, parents facing an ever-increasing threatening culture with aggressive media images, develop a *fait accompli* belief about their teens and substance use. A teen's perception of the harm associated with drug use is constantly being eroded by our culture, which more often than not cultivates a cavalier attitude about marijuana and alcohol. Parents play a significant role when reinforcing a teen's perception that using marijuana and drinking is "harmful."

I think this question also gives parents an opportunity to reflect on their own teen years through the eyes of their own teen. Ask yourself, "What did you need when you were a teen that would have made a difference?" In Michael Riera's book *Uncommon Sense for Parents with Teenagers*, the author emphasizes that parents should have a conversation about alcohol and other drugs and they should examine how they are modeling their relationships with alcohol and other drugs. What you are modeling matters a lot!

In a survey conducted by the Partnership for a Drug Free America, almost all parents surveyed (98%) stated that they had talked with their kids about alcohol and other drugs. However, fewer than 30% of the teenagers recall the conversation. My personal experience with teenagers in the classroom confirms this phenomenon. Parents play a crucial role in educating their kids about the dangers of marijuana and other drugs.

The same survey revealed that teenagers were twice as likely to use pot if they had not learned about the risks from their parents. Both points highlighted in this survey confirm the essential role of open, proactive and transparent communication between parents and children. It also confirms that the communication needs to be ongoing and respond to the developmental and social changes in teenagers.

I was recently at a small private boarding school in New England conducting a parent meeting. It was a typically evening; parents are invited to attend an evening session from 7-8:30 pm or the option of a parent coffee during the day. I presented my typical material and sprinkled the conversation with anecdotes of children I'd met while working. This evening I spoke about Tiffany, a sophomore I met while in Singapore. Tiffany approached me after class in the same kind of sheepish way that most kids with a lot on their mind do—who are unsure of how to say what they really want to say.

Tiffany explained that the group of four to five girls she has known since 7th grade had recently developed a social life that consisted of getting some alcohol and walking up and down Orchard Road; a popular part of downtown Singapore.

Tiffany spoke about the frustration of being a non-user who has to deal with the annoyance and potential danger of intoxicated friends. She explained how unrewarding this experience is for her and how she is getting more and more concerned about her friends. In my experience, Tiffany is unfortunately very common.

Tiffany is a committed non-user who is suffering with that decision going through the transition that is often required as the adjustments and realignments of high school social groups occur when alcohol or other drugs are introduced.

Sophomores in my opinion, experience the most dramatic social turmoil. A good friend calls the sophomore year, "The Perfect Storm" of adolescence. Many educators and parents speak about 8th and 9th grade as key transitional times, and they are, but work long enough with upper school students and you will see the social storm that consumes many sophomores.

Years ago, someone like Tiffany would elicit a typical response from me, "How can I fix this." Here's what usually happened; Tiffany would summon the courage to approach me (and it does take courage); she would express her thoughts, emotions and problem. I would begin to develop solutions to her problem long before she completed her thought and have it ready as soon as she stop talking. It was that at this point that Tiffany's willingness to share would cease; she would get that dazed-over look that indicated "typical adult" and she would scurry away.

I was always left with the feeling that I didn't do anything useful, and you know, I probably didn't.

What I found the be more effective with students experiencing the shifting tides of friendship groups impacted by alcohol and other drug use, is to be present for them, what Alice Walker calls an "empathetic witness". The grief that accompanies the loss and changes in friendships due to alcohol and other drug use is real.

As adults, we can only stand "with" teens as they navigate this time, validate their pain is real, share personal stories about how our friendships have been impacted, and gently remind them that new friends come along, old friendships may rekindle, and that each friendships regardless of term, offers a deep learning we can take with us forever.

Tiffany didn't need my solutions, she already had them; she needed to explore her inner emotional landscape and find her own voice buried beneath the need to be part of and accepted by her peers. Tiffany is engaged in a scenario that is going to repeat itself time and time again throughout her adult life. It has been said by theorist in Women's psychology that Tiffany is facing a female development task, one of being able to separate from relationships that are unfulfilling and toxic. It is a skill I would want all teens to have to take with them into their adult lives.

Tiffany's story sparked an interesting response from a few of the parents who felt I left Tiffany hanging. One parent exclaimed, "what if she went to the other side—and began drinking!" "You could have prevented that by being more assertive and telling other adults at school about her friends!" These parents' responses were motivated by concern of course, but were coming from a parenting belief that we can control people, including our children.

Dr. Thomas Gordon, in his book *Parent Effectiveness Training* says "that most teenage rebellion is a response to ineffective parenting techniques and poor adult communication rather than some natural phenomena that society has come to expect and attach to adolescents."

Far too often in our interaction with kids we use language unintentionally that suggests that they are not equipped with the tools to solve their own problems. We invalidate their feelings as trivial and invalid. My Dad has an expression that for my siblings and I has become infamous for its overall devastating blow to our confidence.

He would say, "Wait until you get into the real world." This little gem was usually reserved for those moments when you were most vulnerable. I remember one day coming home from my summer job in 9th grade. I worked at a local restaurant. I would arrive quite early and wash dishes and pans until the dinner shift during the hottest months of the year. I was proud of the fact that I was a 15 year-old 9th grader who took the initiative to take a full-time job when most of my other friends were working either part-time or not at all.

On a weekly basis, after arriving home and collapsing in a chair, I would attempt to talk about my day with my Dad. I would begin and soon thereafter be hit with the atomic bomb of expressions, "Wait until you get into the real world." I remember thinking, "What world am I living in now? Is there a parallel universe that he's living in that I'm unaware of? As far as I can see, I'm working hard and doing a good job." I love my Dad and he certainly didn't set out to hurt me. But he, like many parents, used language that sent a powerful message such as "what you are feeling is trivial."

Doctor and psychologist, Alfred Adler said when talking about human connection, "When we feel encouraged, we feel capable and appreciated and will generally act in a connected and cooperative way. When we are discouraged, we may act in unhealthy ways by competing, withdrawing, or giving up. It is in finding ways of expressing and accepting encouragement, respect, and social interest that help us feel fulfilled and optimistic.

Those who subscribe to Adler's theories feel, "a misbehaving child is a discouraged child" and that helping children to feel valued, significant, and competent is often the most effective strategy in coping with difficult child behaviors and equipping a teen to say no to destructive behaviors.

Children rely on their parents to lay down the law and establish boundaries. Many of the non-using students I've met in my work have stated that their parents were a primary reason for saying no to drinking and other drug use. They feared disappointing them and the consequences if they broke house rules.

I met Stacey at a school in Massachusetts. Stacey approached me after class to discuss her boyfriend's pot smoking. Eventually our conversation led to talking about her own use of marijuana. "I've smoked pot a few times, but I sing and I don't want the pot smoking to interfere with that. I wonder sometimes what I'd be doing with pot if I didn't sing." Stacey is a good example of how a protective factor (singing) can trump the continuation of a potentially harmful behavior. Parents can learn from this by understanding the need for having kids participate in activities that are nurturing to their emotional well-being.

Being a teen that doesn't use alcohol and other drugs, and I will also suggest a teen that may have tried, but discontinued any regular use, is hard. We live in a culture that says yes. Helping teens navigate through the teen years without being harmed by drug use requires constant vigilance. It means laying down the law of curfews, setting boundaries, being the bad guy (for them), and keeping an open heart and radiating love while doing this.

Teens need to know you love them more than you hate their mistakes. It is possible to raise a drug-free teen or a teen that is free of the harms associated with alcohol misuse and other drug use. It is not a lottery that some parents win and others do not. Is there a little luck involved? Ok, sure. But it is also conscious commitment to a set of beliefs and behaviors that my professional experience and research strongly suggests works.

You can do it! I know you can. And, whether it feels this way or not, your teen is relying on you to come through for them.

CHAPTER 12

How do I start a conversation with my daughter about alcohol and drugs?

The web site www.drugstrategies.org offers the opening statements listed below. However, I think the media and our general culture give us ample opportunities to talk with our kids. I strongly encourage parents to become sensitive to the television and radio and remain so while your children are of school age. Look for television programs that promote health-damaging behavior and ask for your child's feedback. "Hey, what you do think of that?"

You are not the only source of information. This may sound a little self-promoting, but ask your school if they have a prevention program (if they do not, have them call me!). Is it science-based and conducted by a professional with a mental health background. I'd also like to see more families get their health professional involved in prevention. Ask your family doctor or physician's assistant (PA) if during the last check-up they asked your son or daughter about substance use or gave them any prevention material.

How parents can begin the discussion:

> ➤ "I'm troubled by some things I've been reading about smoking, drinking, and other drug use by

people your age. So, it would help me to know what you think about this."
- "It was good we had this chance to watch that program on drug and alcohol abuse together. Some of the scenes bothered me and some of the facts scared me. I'd really like to know what you think about all this."
- "I saw the article about the drug education program in your school newsletter. I'd like to hear more about it, and I'd like to know how you felt about taking part in it."
- Sometimes young people find it difficult to talk with their parents about what worries them, frightens them, or makes them angry. I want you to know that I really would like you to talk with me about these things, and we can always make time to do it. I'm always ready to listen."
- Sometimes young people need to talk with someone outside the family about what's happening with them and their friends. I hope you have an adult you can talk to besides me. If you don't, maybe we can think of someone."[7]

Suggestions for starting a conversation with your children about alcohol and/or other drugs:

- Plan what you want to say. Don't wing it.
- Tell them how you feel, not what you think.
- Set aside the desire to appear cool—be genuine and honest.
- Do not confuse honest with full disclosure.
- Avoid debate and disagreements.
- Listen!

---

[7] http://www.drugstrategies.org retrieved on October 11, 2003

If parents have not built a history of spending time and discussing the small things with their kids, then creating time for the sole purpose of talking about drugs (a big thing) will probably feel awkward. Do it anyway.

Recommended reading:

Faber, A., & Mazlish, E., (1980). *How to talk so kids will listen & listen so kids will talk.* New York, NY: Avon Books, Inc.

CHAPTER 13

How might I teen-proof our house from drugs and alcohol? I'm concerned my teen might take advantage of drinking when I am away.

As the drug educator, I choose to be, who has worked with thousands of teens and the adults in their lives—parents and teachers—one of my goals is to break through some of your old thinking perhaps about drinking when you were younger or maybe the drinking that you saw when you were younger.

Today's contemporary drinking scene is very different in many ways than what we grew up with, but one of the striking ways is the legal and financial consequences of kids drinking today, and the impact it has on their families.

Your home may be a place full of risks, and in this next section we talk about how to make your home safe. In their book, *Parenting 911*, authors Charlene Giannetti and Margaret Sagarese encourage parents to, in their words, teen-proof their home. I could not agree with them more and will offer some of my own suggestions.

Most teenagers will tell you that alcohol is easy to get to. What is surprising is where they get it from. Can you guess? That's right, adults.

According to a study of the American Medical Association, two out of three teens say it's easy to get alcohol from their home without the parents knowing it, one-third of teens say they can get alcohol from their own consenting parents—that we'll talk about later, two out of five teens say it's easy to get alcohol from a friend's parent, and believe it or not, one in four teenagers have been at a party where they were drinking right in front of adults.

Okay, so here are some suggestions that may lower the risks in your home:

- Clean out the medicine cabinet. Discard old prescriptions and keep current medications like your Ritalin or opiates (opiates would be things like Vicodin and Oxycontin) accounted for and secure.

- Do an alcohol inventory. I know this sounds silly but account for all the alcohol in your home, not what's just in the bar, but what may be stored in the basement or the extra refrigerator in the garage. Don't just eyeball that half empty bottle of Vodka but go make sure it's Vodka and not water that's been refilled.

- Avoid buying aerosol cans if an alternative is available to reduce the risk of inhalant abuse.

- Go through your basement or workbench area and secure paint supplies, aerosols, glues, and adhesives that may be huffed.

- Secure in a private place all spare family keys to the home, summer home, vehicles, boats, ATVs, whatever could be used when you're away for the weekend, or your whole family is away; and maybe your son or daughter decides to give one of those spare keys to a friend to use the home.

➢ Install smoke detectors in your child's room and check the batteries from time to time.

➢ Remove all computers from private areas to reduce the risk of children going to web sites and conducting business that is, you know, "sketchy."

➢ And what I consider a great idea—shared with me by a parent at school—was to consider a blackout time for all cell phone activity. This mother had three children with cell phones, and she decided that when she walked into a room at 10 and 11 o'clock at night and the kids were pounding away text messaging, that was it. So she decided 8 o'clock was the blackout time. All cell phones were shut off and turned in, and re-collected each morning. I think that was a great protective idea.

➢ If you're going away for the weekend, consider notifying neighbors and your local police department—if you feel comfortable letting them know that you will be away for the weekend, and if they have the time to drop by and take a look in at the home.

These are just some ideas that may lower the risk in your home.

CHAPTER 14

What do I say to my graduating senior about college next year and all the drinking and partying that I read about in the news?

There's good news and bad news. The bad is that those students drinking on college campuses are drinking more. However, the good news is there is an increase in students who abstain completely from alcohol or drink moderately.

Additional good news is more and more colleges are taking the issue of underage drinking and alcohol abuse seriously. Higher education is developing comprehensive prevention strategies that are making a difference like Social Norms, Brief Interventions, and Motivational Interviewing—see below.

Any parent who reads the newspaper or watches the news has seen and heard tragic stories about dangerous drinking on college campuses. Parents are frightened by these stories and have every right to be. Because of this fear, I have seen a growing myth gain dangerous traction as a parent strategy.

What is this myth?

More parents believe that allowing their high school senior a little rope regarding their drinking will give them the experience to practice safe and responsible drinking in college.

Let me be unequivocal here, this parent strategy is not a good idea and can have dire consequences. My professional experience as well as the research on college drinking does not support this hypothesis to be true.

The big question that I've spent my career thinking about is how do we prepare teens for a world that is filled with alcohol use and abuse with the internal skills that allow them to make safe and responsible decisions. Knowing that every teen and every family is different from the perspective of genetic makeup and social and emotional environments, I have to generalize.

What I have seen and research supports, is a no use message regarding alcohol use—as long as you can maintain it and have significant influence on your teen's decision to drink or abstain. I say significant influence because while your teen is in high school you can have that amount of influence and should maintain it.

Yes, it's true, you lose control when they go to college, but while they are in your home during high school, why not maintain the healthiest standards possible that show the best outcomes? No use is considered the best choice.

College Parents of America (CPA) shares the concern of dangerous drinking in college. CPA is advising parents to talk with their children during summer breaks about the impact of binge drinking. College Parents of America encourages parents to take time in summer to speak with their students about alcohol and offers the following eight talking points.

1. **Set clear and realistic expectations regarding academic performance.**
Studies conducted nationally have demonstrated that partying may contribute as much to a student's decline in grades as the difficulty of his or her academic work. If students know their parents expect sound academic work, they are likely to be more devoted to their studies and have less time to get in trouble with alcohol.

2. **Stress to students that alcohol is toxic and excessive consumption can be fatal.** This is not a scare tactic. The fact is students die every year from alcohol poisoning. Discourage dangerous drinking through participation in drinking games, fraternity hazing, or in any other way. Parents should ask their students to also have the courage to intervene when they see someone putting their life at risk through participation in dangerous drinking.

3. **Tell students to intervene when classmates are in trouble with alcohol**. Nothing is more tragic than an unconscious student being left to die while others either fail to recognize that the student is in jeopardy or fail to call for help due to fear of getting the student in trouble.

4. **Tell students to stand up for their right to a safe academic environment.** Students who do not drink can be affected by the behavior of those who do, ranging from interrupted study time to assault or unwanted sexual advances. Students can confront these problems directly by discussing them with the offender. If that fails, they should notify the housing director or other residence hall staff.

5. **Know the alcohol scene on campus and talk to students about it.** Students grossly exaggerate the use of alcohol and other drugs by their peers. A recent survey found that University of Oregon students believed 96 percent of their peers drink alcohol at least once a week, when the actual rate was 52 percent. Students are highly influenced by peers and tend to drink up to what they perceive to be the norm. Confronting misperceptions about alcohol use is vital.

6. **Avoid tales of drinking exploits from your own college years.** Entertaining students with stories of drinking back in "the good old days" normalizes what, even then, was abnormal behavior. It also appears to give parental approval to dangerous alcohol consumption.

7. **Encourage your student to volunteer in community work.** In addition to structuring free time, volunteerism provides students with opportunities to develop job-related skills and to gain valuable experience. Helping others also gives students a broader outlook and a healthier perspective on the opportunities they enjoy. Volunteer work on campus helps students further connect with their school, increasing the likelihood of staying in college.

8. **Make it clear—Underage alcohol consumption and driving after drinking are against the law**. Parents should make it clear that they do not condone breaking the law. Parents of college students should openly and clearly express disapproval of underage drinking and dangerous alcohol consumption. And, if parents themselves drink, they should present a positive role model in the responsible use of alcohol.

Above all ASK QUESTIONS!

You have a right to know that a college is serious in its efforts to address dangerous drinking and other drug-related problems. Here are questions provided by the US Department of Education Safe and Drug-Free Schools Program and the Higher Education Center for Alcohol and Other Drug Prevention. You should expect college officials to answer these questions with hard evidence to support their claims.

- What steps has the college president taken to provide visible, consistent leadership on this issue?
- Does the college have a clearly defined alcohol and other drug policy? What is it? What are the consequences for infractions?
- Will the administration inform parents if a student is disciplined or arrested for alcohol or other drug related infractions, or hospitalized for drug or alcohol use?
- What percent of students join fraternities or sororities? What is the school doing to reduce alcohol use among these groups, whose members tend to drink more heavily than others?
- What proportion of the athletics budget comes from the alcohol industry? (Accepting such money sends a mixed message to students.)
- What training do residential advisers have in identifying and helping students who may have alcohol or other drug problems?
- What percent of students are involved in community service? (Students who are involved in such activities tend to have fewer alcohol—and other drug-related problems.)
- What treatment and other services are available for students who have alcohol and other drug-related problems?

During school breaks and summer, talk with your student about alcohol. While parents may not be able to actively monitor students away from home, they can be available to talk and listen, and that is just as important. It can do more than help shape lives; it can save lives.

Recommended reading and websites:

Wechsler PhD, H, & Wuethrich, B., (2002) *Dying to Drink: Confronting Binge Drinking on College Campuses*

http://.collegeparents.org

http://www.harvardsph.org

*See Social Norms in Defining Terms

CHAPTER 15

Where do kids get the alcohol? And when do kids start drinking or using other drugs?

Most kids will tell you they get alcohol from a friend's home (parent's supply). Others will say they have an older sibling or family member buy it for them. In a study by the Center for Addiction and Substance Abuse (CASA)[8], 95% of 12th graders, 28% of 10th graders, and 18% of 8th graders said alcohol was easy to get. The top four means where adolescents get there alcohol is through some form of adult interaction.

Compliant adults are those who go out and purchase alcohol for their minor child and friends usually under the mindset that it is better that they are drinking in an environment where they can be supervised. Even if this were true, and I do not believe in this strategy. There are plenty of stories where teens who have been drinking in this "supervised" environment leave the home undetected and get injured or worse, die, in some alcohol-related accident.

Non-compliant adults are those who's alcohol supply has been raided. Adults with teens should begin to think more

---

[8] National Survey of American Attitudes on Substance Abuse XVI: Teens and Parents (CASA study, August 2011)

seriously about the amounts of alcohol in the home and how the supply is monitored. When thinking about adults, we often think of parents, and people in the 30's, 40's or 50's.

But in every town, there are those people in their early 20's who for whatever reason have not moved on with their lives and still make up their social lives by hanging around with the high school crowd. These young adults pose a serious danger due to their legal status which allows them to purchase alcohol.

Last, but not least, is the returning college student, perhaps an older sibling, who has secured a fake ID at college. The market for fake IDs is alive and well. All parents must have a serious conversation with their older children about purchasing alcohol for the minor siblings.

Limiting the access that teens have to alcohol and other drugs is an important prevention strategy for parents and community leaders. During the middle school years is a time when parents should be thinking about securing their alcohol supply if they have one and/or becoming more conscious of how much they have. It is not about not trusting your child. It is about helping them avoid any potential pressures a friend may put on them to access it.

All parents should be aware and thinking about safety around the three cabinets; gun, liquor, and medicine.

According to recent data, the age of first use of alcohol and other drugs has dropped to near 13 years of age. I know it is hard to imagine your middle schooler—who not too long ago was mostly occupied with innocent social activities—being exposed to alcohol and other drugs. Even harder to imagine is that they may say yes to an offer. I don't want any parent to become riddled with panic and anxiety.

However, it is smart to begin to make room for the idea that your young son or daughter may be exposed to substances. It is worth bringing up at this age level and having an ongoing awareness and openness to the issue. You'd be laying the ground for a transparency of some degree for years to come that could make all the difference in high school and college and adulthood.

Imagine them thanking you for empowering them to make better choices earlier. Imagine them perpetuating this kind of parenting with their own children? What possibilities are you interested in causing?

CHAPTER 16

Should I allow my son to go to a party where I know there will be drinking? He tells me he doesn't drink when he's there and I believe him, but I'm not sure if I should let him go. He says it's the only fun thing to do.

It is a little sad that he feels it's the only fun thing to do. I think the community you live in needs to look at that statement and ask itself whether that's true. Many people who work with youth will tell you that there are indeed less appropriate opportunities and places for teenagers to "hang out" and have fun than there were years ago.

However, I guess I don't know what he means by fun thing to do. He says he doesn't drink so does he mean it is fun to be around drunk people? I don't recall during my early days of sobriety enjoying being around drunk people very much.

Most high school students tell me the same. Does he mean hanging out with his non-drinking friends at the party is fun? If that's the case, he can do that at your house can't he? So, maybe we have to make room for the idea that he may be drinking and going to this party is not a great idea.

It's a tough call. We all want our children to be socially successful. Parents are fooling themselves if they don't believe some of their own childhood "stuff" is not tied up in their children's social success. We may be older, but we all remember what the social scene was like in high school.

The question is what you are willing to tolerate and gamble for that social success. Here is clue you've negotiated a bad deal. If you are still waiting up around the time of curfew, staring out the window until you see his car, and when you do, you breathe a deep sigh of relief—you've got a bad deal. Negotiating win-win deals with your children does not mean their needs get met at the expense of yours.

Educator and trainer Jane Bluestein suggests that next time your son hits you with the "It's the only fun thing to do!" speech, calmly say, "You know, going to a party where there's drinking, doesn't work for me."

Stay silent. Allow your son to renegotiate until you've found a social activity that works for both of you.

CHAPTER 17

I heard the pot smoked today is 10-20 times stronger than the pot that was smoked a generation ago? Is that true?

The simple answer is yes. That being said, I heard conflicting stories about this. One story says that pot is stronger today because of better growing methods. This makes sense to me considering the economics of marijuana. Another story suggests it is only mildly stronger, let's say about 4-5% stronger, not 20-30% like you've suggested.

According to the federal Potency Monitoring Project, in 1985, the average THC content of commercial-grade marijuana was 2.84%, and the average for high-grade sensimilia in 1985 was 7.17%. In 1995, the potency for commercial-grade marijuana averaged 3.73%, while the potency of sinsemilla in 1995 averaged 7.51%. In 2001, commercial-grade marijuana averaged 4.72% THC, and the potency of sinsemilla in 2001 averaged 9.03%.[9] The Cannabis Potency Monitoring Project, sponsored by the

---

[9] Quarterly Report #76, Nov. 9, 2001 – Feb. 8, 2002, Table 3, p. 8, University of Mississippi Potency Monitoring Project (Oxford, MS: National Center for the Development of Natural Products, Research Institute of Pharmaceutical Sciences, 2002), Mahmoud A. ElSohly, PhD, Director, NIDA Marijuana Project (NIDA Contract #N01DA – 0 – 7707).

National Institute of Drug Abuse (NIDA) and conducted by the Research Institute of Pharmaceutical Sciences tracks changes in the delta-9-tetrahydrocannabinol (THC) content (potency) of cannabis (marijuana, hashish, hashish oil) seized in the United States shows only modest increases in marijuana and sensimilia.

I think there are more important trends occurring here than the potency of marijuana. What is really scary to me is the age of first use has declined year after year. Your average pot smoker in the 1960's was well into her late teens or early college years when they first used marijuana.

Today, the average first-time user is in the eighth grade, and the age seems to be dropping every few years. Regardless of potency, there is a huge difference between the social, emotional, and psychological resilience of an eighth grader and an eighteen year old. Personally, I'd rather not see either smoke pot. However, I see that as the bigger, more confirmable trend than the pot potency debate.

The National Institute for Drug Abuse (NIDA) has stated for years that for each year a teenagers delays their relationship with alcohol and other drugs, their risk of addiction lowers by 14%.

The debate of whether pot is stronger today is moot for another reason that is inherent in the way pot smokers use marijuana. Unlike alcohol, where users will continue to drink well past their limits, pot smokers tend to stop smoking pot once they have achieve the desired state of marijuana intoxication. For this reason, the potency debate loses some of its strength because regardless of potency, drug use is ceased once the drugs effects are achieved.

I don't think the pot in the 1960's or 1970's caused less neurological damage than the pot today. I do believe we know more about adolescent neurological development today which makes what we always knew scarier and more real.

CHAPTER 18

I've been to a million of these parent education workshops, but the parents that really need to be here are not. How do we get them to show up? I'm tired of picking up the pieces from these parents.

I hear this at almost every parent meeting. Where are those parents? You know, the ones serving and buying the booze for kids. Those parents who are having parties, allowing our children to drink in a "safe" environment, going to bed and not checking on them! Where are they? They're home watching TV right now, not giving a second thought to our concerns. They don't see their actions as a problem. They probably think we are being unrealistic and naïve.

Unfortunately, they will always be there, in every community, undermining the hard work we are doing and putting kids at risk. A young man I met at a school in St. Paul said to me recently, "It only takes one or two of those parents to destroy a community."

A question I'm often asked is, "With all the programming targeted at kids and alcohol, why have we seen little or sometimes no improvement in the level of alcohol and other drug use?"

I think the primary reason is that we focus too much of our attention on kids! I think it is time to speak frankly. I don't think we can afford to wait for these parents to see the light and finally decide that they'll come to a parent meeting.

Heads of School and PA (Parent Association) leaders need to consider implementing mandatory meetings for parents of children coming to their school. Not every year, but every parent with a child at that school must attend a parent education series that talks about the physical, emotional, psychological, and legal dangers of underage drinking.

We need to get more creative in reaching parents. There is a growing interest in using web-based learning tools to reach parents. I think we need to continue to use active parent education experiences like workshops like these and interesting speakers. However, not all parents are interested in attending a workshop or have the schedule to do so. For that reason, we need to look at more effective passive educational campaigns.

Social norms marketing strategies have shown promise in affecting attitudes and beliefs about alcohol and other drugs. We need to customize educational pieces for parents that really catch their attention. An organization I like called The Parent Party Patrol has put together parent educational material, which I think is very appealing and useful for parents.

Touch. Inspire. Motivate.

CHAPTER 19

Don't you think you are sending the wrong message to kids when you are a recovering person teaching drug education?

I'm assuming by your question that you mean am I giving teens the impression that drugs aren't that bad because I've recovered and I'm leading a productive life?

I think the point of being sick, as the state of addiction is often described, is to get well. I'm not apologetic about getting well or leading a productive life with strong relationships and financial independence. My recovering is work, ongoing work, which is something I point out to teens. The work of recovery and subsequent consequences—which is more peace of mind for friends and family—should be the goal of recovery.

I think you have a right to be concerned about a recovering person teaching prevention. I understand the concern; perhaps it is like going to a dentist with bad teeth. There is also research that suggests that recovering people perpetuate the myth that everyone is doing it (drugs).

However, recovering people teaching prevention can be a very powerful strategy, especially when the instructor understands his or her personal narrative around their addictive experience and can translate it into meaningful education.

I think it is very important for a student who may have a friend or relative struggling with an addiction to see a person who has put the addiction into remission, to see that when a person receives effective treatment they can recover and lead productive lives.

All too often, we present drug addiction as a lifetime sentence of misery, when in fact; it is not for most people who have had an addiction. This doesn't mean it should dilute the message to teens regarding the dangers of dangerous drinking and other drug use. There are serious consequence to alcohol misuse and other drug use.

I do not think being is recovery is itself a prerequisite for teaching drug education. It may be an added benefit, but being in recovery is not a skill associated with facilitating drug education seminars. It is a condition of the person that may or may not have value. Drug educators who do their jobs well have years of experience and training to engage students, faculty, parents, and administrators in a shared vision of drug-free and harm-free living from substances. It is a mistake to assume that being is recovery allows you to be in the room. That alone is not enough. I think of myself as an educator who happens to be recovering from the experience of addiction, rather than an addict who educates.

I truly hope that the students, parents, teachers, administrators and community members I work with really get that I care deeply about the message I bring, the work I do and the impact I desire to make in my lifetime. Can you appreciate that?

CHAPTER 20

My daughter's prom is coming up. My wife and I are worried about the whole party scene surrounding the prom. What can we do to ensure she has a great time but safely?

What is it about a prom or graduation that makes rational parents go bonkers?

As we move into the prom and graduation season, many parents and school officials worry about the safety of their children. A Google search under the term "Safe Prom" turned up hundreds of sites that focus on encouraging students to make safe and healthy choices. There were schools conducting pre-prom events showing the dangers of drinking and driving and many web sites promoting limos and clothing.

However, there were few if any sites encouraging or guiding parents to take the lead role in creating a safe prom night.

For the past fifteen years, I've worked as a drug education specialist in secondary schools educating principals, headmasters, parents, and students about the dangers of underage drinking and other drug use. When conversation turns to a horror story about prom night or graduation party disasters, in many cases, it is a parent who has either rented a hotel room with little or no supervision or purchased the alcohol consumed.

A 2002 study revealed that 40% of teen traffic fatalities during the prom and graduation weekends were alcohol-related. Fatal car accidents, injuries, and assaults are not an adolescent rite of passage for any child. Underage drinking is a major factor in the two leading causes of teenage deaths: car crashes and fatal injuries. Alcohol abuse is also linked to two-thirds of sexual assaults and date rapes of teens, and increases the likelihood of unsafe and unplanned sexual activity. According to the American College of Preventive Medicine, approximately 75% of adolescent morbidity and mortality is associated with behavioral health risks, of which a large portion can be attributed to alcohol and other drug use.

Under the new social host law, many states are prosecuting parents who serve alcohol to minors. Ohio has a program called "Parents Who Host Lose the Most." Here in Massachusetts, not a month goes by without a courtroom appearance by a parent for serving alcohol to a minor.

Schools, law enforcement, and parent associations need to reach out to parents and educate them about the legal and financial risks of serving alcohol to minors and renting hotel rooms to minors under their name during the upcoming prom and graduation event.

The prom and graduation are celebrations full of expectation. Each is a meaningful milestone for students and should be celebrated with friends and family. Many students who would normally not drink or engage in sexual behavior are tempted and under more pressure than any other time during the high school years.

Parents need to set appropriate expectations and continue to enforce household rules about drinking and curfews. If parents do their job, the only horror show should be when your teen looks back years from now and says, "Oh my, what was I wearing?" "My hair!!!"

Recommendations for Parents

Do not extend curfews—Teen car crashes and deaths increase exponentially late at night. If you extend curfews, do not give large blocks of unaccounted for time. Know where your children are, how long they will be there, when will they be leaving, who is there, and who is supervising the event.

Do not rent a hotel room—Is anyone really surprised when a tragedy happens after a parent rents a hotel room unsupervised? The parent must be there, not out to dinner with friends or on another floor asleep.

Be up when they come home—My mother once told me that her prevention plan was coffee and lights—be wide awake with the lights on sitting at the kitchen table, coffee in hand, when they come in the front door. A teen's curfew should never exceed the parents' ability to stay up.

Initiate a dialogue about your expectations—Although you may feel you've communicated your desires and consequence for unwanted behaviors many times, the prom and graduation season is a great time to remind your children. Teens who normally would pass on drinking, drug use, or sexual behavior are tempted in ways they are usually not during the rest of the year. Talk to them about drinking and driving, getting in the car with drunk drivers, and what they can do if something goes unexpectedly wrong. Consider role-playing a few scenarios. Research points to parents who discuss possible scenarios in great detail and seek their teens' knowledge about what to do increase the chances of their teen actually doing what they suggest.

Keep the party local—Don't be tempted to allow your children to celebrate at a beach or other remote location. Allowing your teen to take off to a remote location with little supervision creates unnecessary risk.

The prom is a rite of passage that your teen should enjoy and remember for a lifetime. The following are talking points and should be part of your family's prom preparation:

- Talk with your teen. How are they feeling about the prom? What is your teen most excited about? What is your teen most nervous about?
- Who is your teen's date and/or group of friends with whom they will be attending the prom? Does your teen know them well? Do you? What are the conversations you need to have based on the age, values and beliefs of your teen and this group?
- Have you met and do you know the parents of your teen's date and prom group?

CHAPTER 21

My son is curious about alcohol. Should I sit down with him and allow him to drink until he knows how it feels to be drunk to eliminate the curiosity? My father did this with me and I didn't have any problems.

This question is fresh in my mind because I just returned from a parent meeting where a parent asked this question. There is a tendency or can I say strong desire from parents to hear the "right" answer to these questions. Unfortunately, there are no simple right answers when you are dealing with human behavior—especially adolescents.

One person may react one way and another just the opposite. My mother always said that there were many constants when parenting her kids, one of those constants was that every one of her children needed a different approach.

Knowing that there are no certainties, research has assisted educators in choosing strategies that have higher probabilities of success. I believe this question highlights the shortsightedness of parents to wish that the risk for alcohol and other drug use boils down to curiosity only. It doesn't. The issue is multidimensional.

I believe experimentation with alcohol is in some aspects a final process in a series of cognitive steps.

I've worked for years in European countries. My initial impression was that alcohol would not be a big deal over there. With the lower and oftentimes non-existent drinking age, the appeal to drink would be less intense. During a class with mixed group of teenagers from all over Europe I asked about the drinking scene. They began to tell me about how American teenagers were craziest with the alcohol and did not know how to pace themselves.

That aside, I asked, "How many of you are concerned about a friend's alcohol use?" Almost a third of the hands were raised. Alcohol may be viewed differently by European youth and their parents. But alcohol still causes the same harm to social, cognitive, and neurological development of European teenagers as American teenagers.

CHAPTER 22

Is it okay to drink in front of my kids?

I have not read any research that suggests it is harmful to drink in front of your kids. Anecdotally, I have heard many professionals proclaim that if parents were serious about raising drug-free children then they would abstain from drinking until their children were of the age to drink. I think that's ridiculous.

Kids are bombarded with images of people drinking abusively and self-medicating in many other ways, what could be better than to provide your children with an appropriate model of moderate and responsible drinking—assuming you do drink. I have asked kids this question directly. Most adolescents believe it is okay for their parents to drink as long as they do it responsibly. I do not know if drinking in front of your children is harmful.

I do know that adolescents are very aware of how much you drink and why you drink. They are also very aware if your action matches your talk about the issue. For instance, if you believe drinking and driving is dangerous (I hope you do) then do you back up that belief by making sure that you do not have a few cocktails and then drive the family home from the restaurant. You may be below the legal limit and you may quite capable of driving, however, what message are you sending?

How about handing the keys to your spouse as you leave the restaurant so your kids can see you doing it? What message is that sending? I saw a commercial on TV this year that showed a man arriving at a party with his favorite six-pack of beer. He got out of his car, pulled out a knife and punctured all his tires! The commercial ended by saying, enjoy the beer and never drink and drive.

Is that what it takes to make a responsible decision? How alcohol is used in your home is a personal choice by all families. I think care has to be given to the "meaning" attached to alcohol use when adolescents reach the age of awareness.

A mother shared a story of her seventh grader who commented on the empty bottle of wine in the trash on Friday. She said, "My son said, hey mom I noticed that you bought that bottle on Monday and it is empty now?"

How might you respond if this were happening to you? Remember, actions speak louder than words. And if you think your kids aren't seeing what is going on, think again.

Some Final Words

"Just This Weekend"

I was in Chattanooga giving a parent meeting. I was telling the story of a young lady I met years ago in St. Paul. She was a sophomore who was participating in one of my seminars. I was eating lunch alone one day and she joined me.

We began talking about her social life and the whole drinking scene in school. She said, "You know, parents can be so naive. They like to think my kids went through D.A.R.E. or an intense middle school health program, so now you don't have to worry about anything."

I asked her, "So what's the real deal? What are we adults missing?" "What you're missing is that the decision to drink or not to drink for a lot of kids is weekend by weekend."

I asked, "Well how do you decide if you will or won't? "There are a lot of factors. I take athletics seriously so that affects my decision, or if I'm not feeling well, and sometimes I'm just not in the mood to drink. But ultimately it comes down to mom and dad."

"What do you mean, I asked?" "It's simple. If I get the sense that they're on top of things that weekend, for instance, they'll be up when I come home, or they're doing the whole calling ahead thing or checking up on me, then I'm out. The decision is made for me. But if they look tired and I know they're crashing or they don't get too nosey about my plans, then the door is definitely open. "

A mother in the front row had a facial expression that could only be interpreted as being overwhelmed. I asked her "Are you okay? It's so much, she said. My daughter is in the ninth grade; I've got four maybe five years of this in front of me. Many parents in the room voiced agreement.

I said, "You know if you think about this as four or five years, then yes it will produce fear, anxiety, and feelings of being overwhelmed. I have found that if I focus on what's next, and doing that task well, then things get a little easier to manage. Focus on what you need to do just this weekend."

After that parent meeting I continued to use "just this weekend" to end many of my parent meetings. Each week I'd start adding what I thought were some tasks or affirmations to the "just this weekend" phrase. At the time I said it, I didn't realize that "just this weekend" had a lot in common with a simple yet profound wisdom of another phrase, "one day at a time", which has had a powerful impact on millions of people trying to stay clean and sober in 12-step programs.

I'd like to share with you the Just This Weekend: A Parent's Pledge:

"Just This Weekend"

Just this weekend, I will call ahead to where you are going to make sure the environment is safe.

I will sometimes ask tough and embarrassing questions to ensure your safety.

I may show up to where you are to ensure that you're there doing what you said.

I will be awake when you come home at night to ensure you are safe and not under the influence of alcohol or other drugs.

I will be your parent; this means you may dislike me sometimes.

I will be your parent; this may mean saying no to your wants.

I will not confuse my wants with your needs.

Just this weekend, I will try my best to take care of myself emotionally, physically, and spiritually so I can take care of you.

Just this weekend.

To learn more about Jeff Wolfsberg, his work as a keynote speaker, facilitator and his training programs, please visit www.jeffwolfsberg.com.

Resources

Faces & Voices of Recovery
A national nonprofit organization working to mobilize, organize and rally Americans in a campaign to end discrimination, broaden understanding and achieve a just response to addiction.
www.facesandvoicesofrecovery.org

Harm Reduction Coalition
A national advocacy group that promotes programs to tackle adverse effects of drug abuse, such as overdose, HIV, hepatitis C, addiction, and incarceration.
www.harmreduction.org

Join Together
A Boston University School of Health project supporting effective drug and alcohol policy and providing information on current policy and legislative issues, political advocacy, and a large online database and documents library.
www.jointogether.org

National Association for Children of Alcoholics (NACoA)
An organization advocating for children and families affected by alcoholism and other drug dependencies.
www.nacoa.org

Partnership for a Drug-Free America
A nonprofit coalition of scientists, communications professionals and parenting experts seeking to reduce demand for drugs through anti-drug advertising and other forms of media communication.
www.drugfreeamerica.org

Marijuana Anonymous
A program to help people recover from marijuana addiction.
www.marijuana-anonymous.org

Narcotics Anonymous (NA)
An international association of recovering drug addicts.
www.na.org

Alcoholics Anonymous (AA)
The world's leading 12-step fellowship, designed to help people overcome drinking problems.
www.aa.org

Cocaine Anonymous
A program to help people recover from cocaine addiction.
www.ca.org

Co-Dependents Anonymous
A program that helps people with codependency problems to learn to form healthier relationships.
www.coda.org

Sex and Love Addicts Anonymous
A program helping people with sex and love addictions.
www.slaafws.org

Higher Education Center for Alcohol and Other Drug Prevention
An organization funded by the US Department of Education that supports higher education institutions in trying to address alcohol and other drug problems.
www.higheredcenter.org

Brown Center for Alcohol and Addiction Studies
A department at Brown University that promotes the prevention, and treatment of alcohol and other drug use problems through research, education, training and policy advocacy.
www.caas.brown.edu

Children of Alcoholics Foundation
A nonprofit organization that provides educational materials and services to help professionals, children, and adults dealing with parental addiction.
www.coaf.org

Center for Substance Abuse Prevention
An agency run by the Substance Abuse and Mental Health Services Administration that provides leadership in the federal effort to prevent alcohol, tobacco and other drug problems.
www.samhsa.gov

College Drinking Prevention
A government-supported program that provides strategies and solutions to prevent the harmful consequences of college binge drinking.
www.cadca.org

Attachment & Trauma Network
A network that provides advocacy, support and education and about the most important dynamic in child development: the attachment relationship with adults. An especially important resource for people working with kids who have experienced trauma.
http://www.attachtrauma.org/education.html

The Landmark Forum
A powerful and effective weekend course in personal growth and transformation, available internationally. I can attest from personal experience and observation that the program's efficacy in empowering people to dissolve old patterns, hidden beliefs and ways of being, and in creating richer and more fulfilling lives and relationships, is unparalleled.
http://www.landmarkforum.com

For a more comprehensive list of resources, please visit http://www.jeffwolfsberg.com

www.ingramcontent.com/pod-product-compliance
Lightning Source LLC
LaVergne TN
LVHW051501070426
835507LV00022B/2867